MORE HARM THAN GOOD

MORE HARM
THAN GOOD

WHAT YOUR DOCTOR MAY NOT TELL YOU
ABOUT COMMON TREATMENTS AND PROCEDURES

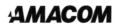

ALAN ZELICOFF, M.D. and MICHAEL BELLOMO

₁AMACOM

AMERICAN MANAGEMENT ASSOCIATION

New York • Atlanta • Brussels • Chicago • Mexico City • San Francisco •
Shanghai • Tokyo • Toronto • Washington, D. C.

Special discounts on bulk quantities of AMACOM books are available to corporations, professional associations, and other organizations. For details, contact Special Sales Department, AMACOM, a division of American Management Association, 1601 Broadway, New York, NY 10019.
Tel: 212-903-8316. Fax: 212-903-8083.
E-mail: specialsls@amanet.org
Website: www.amacombooks.org/go/specialsales
To view all AMACOM titles go to: www.amacombooks.org

This publication is designed to provide accurate and authoritative information in regard to the subject matter covered. It is sold with the understanding that the publisher is not engaged in rendering legal, accounting, or other professional service. If legal advice or other expert assistance is required, the services of a competent professional person should be sought.

Library of Congress Cataloging-in-Publication Data

Zelicoff, Alan P.
    More harm than good : what your doctor may not tell you about common treatments and procedures / Alan Zelicoff and Michael Bellomo.
        p. cm.
    Includes bibliographical references and index.
    ISBN-13: 978-0-8144-0027-2
    ISBN-10: 0-8144-0027-2
    1. Medical care—United States—Evaluation.   2. Medical economics.   I. Bellomo, Michael.   II. Title.
    RA399.A3Z45 2008
    338.4'73621—dc22
                                                                    2007049097

Printing number

10 9 8 7 6   5 4 3 2 1

ON OCCASSION, it may appear to the reader that we are too harsh on the medical profession's decision-making abilities. But we recognize that, in the end, all patients are individuals, and the authors would like to dedicate this book in part to the entire hospital staff at Kaiser Permanente in Sacramento, California. Their decisions and prompt actions in early 2000 are the reason for Michael Bellomo being here today to write these words.

Any book that pretends to prescribe solutions to the difficult problem of financing health care while improving quality must do so based in clear science and unbiased analysis. We were first inspired to write this book by the work of John E. Wennberg and colleagues at the Dartmouth Medical School, who have for four decades studied the trends in health care practices across the United States, publishing their findings in the *Dartmouth Atlas of Health Care*, so well known to every manager in the enormous health care industry, but which somehow has escaped the attention of virtually every doctor and nurse practicing medicine. We hope that we can contribute in some small way to widening the audience that hears their message. There is no one—from patient to political decision maker—who will not benefit from the lessons their work has taught us.

CONTENTS

F O R E 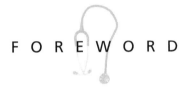 W O R D

"If you always do what you've always done—you'll always get what you've always got."

IF THE CURRENT DISCUSSIONS about the "crisis of the uninsured" remain focused on the mechanisms of payment, we'll continue to have a dysfunctional health care system that fails all our citizenry while squandering monies that are needed for education, infrastructure, and rationale social programs.

This book, *More Harm Than Good*, will make an important contribution to what will inevitably be a post-election national discussion about how we can assure that none among us are denied access to care. It is, in fact, a transformational book that proposes a shift in discourse from the pedantic arguments about mechanisms of payment to discussions that consider the essential question of what services and therapies should be provided to assure that all of our citizens have the health and medical resources they need so they can live productive and fulfilling lives. One of the many unique contributions of this book is the authors' thesis that if we replace rhetoric driven health policy with health policy driven by good science, we'll be able to balance the seemingly uncontrollable inflationary spiral in large part caused by an uncritical acceptance of the products of the evolutionary explosion in biomedical technologies.

This book empowers those of us with chronic diseases to actively participate in the responsibility for the management of our conditions by spelling out the essentials of care standards for the most common conditions. More important, however, the authors put technology and chronic diseases in perspective, and cogently make the point that low technology care often results in far better outcomes at less monetary cost with far less opportunity for harm from unintended consequences. As potential, if not actual patients, all of us should read and heed the admonitions against succumbing to the temptation to jump onto the latest offering from the disease prevention marketers that offer the promise of disease prevention using the latest version of Spock's tricorder. For the authors clearly show the pitfalls and discuss the human wreckage that often lies unacknowledged at the bottom of the slippery slope of screening protocols that have not been subjected to a rigorous scientific validation process. Similarly, the book empowers us to ask our surgeons to spell out the evidence that a proffered procedure has clearly validated indications as well as discussing the probability that the suggested therapeutic procedure will result in a positive outcome and not turn into a potentially crippling therapeutic misadventure.

Far from therapeutic nihilists, the authors continually recognize and pay tribute to the advances afforded by the revolution in biotechnology and bioengineering. At the same time they audaciously recommend that we change the way new technologies are introduced by insisting that each be subjected to carefully designed rigorous validation studies. In fact, one of the most novel contributions of this book is the plea that all practitioners contribute their data to the millions of natural experiments that arise daily from individual patient encounters. The section of the book that outlines how a system using universal medical records in individual practitioners' offices could be used to pool data and rapidly address the pressing and unanswered clinical questions, is itself worth the price of the book.

The authors also address workforce issues, but again in novel and significantly different ways. Out of the recognition that nonphysician providers can and do provide significant volumes of care across the medical spectrum, the authors depart from the usual simplistic calls to increase physician manpower. Instead, they call for an analysis of workforce needs built on the concept of the division of labor, and recognize that rather than produce more physicians, perhaps we should produce more physician assistants and fewer physicians. However important the call for a rational discussion of future work force needs, it pales in comparison to the authors' well-justified call to revise medical education across all disciplines. Their call to replace the elements of education that enhance practice by rote with educational elements that will give future practitioners the skills and abilities to truly practice evidence based medicine is one that truly warrants the attention of curriculum committees in the nation's health science schools. In today's practice environment when more than ever a license to practice is also a license to kill, it is unconscionable that someone could graduate without essential skills to understand and apply the statistics that form the basis of solid, safe, clinical decision making.

This is a book that not only deserves to be read, but its carefully thought prescriptions should be assimilated in the warp and woof of the ensuing health care debate. If I were wealthy, I'd mail a copy to all of the nation's practitioners, health policy wonks, and every voting household in the country.

—William Stanhope, P.A.
School of Public Health
Saint Louis University

INTRODUCTION

IT'S HARD TO PICK UP a newspaper or popular periodical and not read about an exciting new medical breakthrough. Usually the breathlessly worded article recounts the results of a small group of patients with an incurable disease who seem to have been successfully treated—or if not cured, at least helped—by a new medication or surgical procedure. Or perhaps there are remarkable pictures of the inside of the body or images of the brain that show its function changing while people carry on normal tasks. The medical author may go on to quote the researcher studying a new scanner's pictures who speculates that there's little doubt that within a few years the cause of Alzheimer's disease will be revealed due to new tests like the one described in the four-hundred-word article.

But what one almost never sees is the follow-up to those stories. Perhaps the effects of the new treatment were either temporary or had down-the-line side effects that led to what appeared to be a fruitful line of research being abandoned. Maybe the new scanning machine revealed so many apparent abnormalities or gave so much inexplicable information that either no one knew what to do with the data, or worse, acted on it (usually in the hope of helping the patient), but ended up doing little more than proving that the information wasn't worth having in the first place. Meanwhile, many of these scanners might have been bought and installed by people—including physicians—hoping to make a profit. Of course, because the costs are high, even absent any evidence of benefit, they get used—and often paid for by patients directly if insurance companies refuse to do so (and insurance companies are not always wrong in this judgment). Billions of dollars are wasted every year, and, more times than we like to admit, people are harmed.

As we will show in this book, scientifically and economically proven treatments—which save both lives and money—are being underused. At the same time, expensive or invasive procedures and treatments (or those that are both expensive and invasive) are clearly overutilized. In at least the elderly population—where the most suffering occurs—it is now clear that we have gone beyond the law of diminishing returns to the law of *negative* returns. Put another way, from community hospitals to academic medical centers, in both private and public hospitals large and small, there is a better than even chance that the next dollar being spent for medical care is, in fact, *lessening* either the quality of life or longevity. It is highly likely that the same result obtains in doctor's offices and physician-owned hospitals and diagnostic centers.

There is no doubt that many people have been helped by high-tech modern medical advances. The engineering research into new materials has led to long-lasting joint replacements for worn-out hips and knees that otherwise would have been so painful as to render many people with degenerative arthritis immobile, leading in turn to the loss of quality and enjoyment of life and further complications from muscle atrophy and bone thinning due to lack of use. Who among us now expects to give up walking for enjoyment or for countless activities of daily living as we age? Similar work in physics and engineering have led to lens replacements for cataracts, once an almost inevitable result of aging and a certain decline into blindness. With a 20-minute procedure, sight is now restored, and the implantation of artificial lenses gives many people in their seventies and eighties better sight than they enjoyed when they were 40. Few of us will ever suffer for long from cataracts when we live into old age.

And, for a small number of people, the miracles of organ transplantation—first of kidneys, then hearts, and now livers and lungs—have completely reversed various chronic, otherwise irreparable damage to these organs and eliminated the attendant suffering and inevitable decline until death supervenes. This is a tiny percentage of the population, to be sure, but we have no doubt that the individuals and those who care about them would say that the benefits were worth the cost (and sometimes the long recovery periods).

At the same time, ask most Americans if they are satisfied with their health care and you'll find that the answer is mostly no. As with any polling, the answer depends very much on the way the question is asked and also *who* is asked. In 2003, among the fewer and fewer Americans with employer-provided health insurance, more than 80% rated their health care plan or coverage positively,[1] but more than half are worried that coverage either will be unaffordable or vastly different (and unsatisfactory) in the future. By 2007, just four years later, in a Zogby poll only about 58% of Americans—most still covered by either employer-paid insurance or, if elderly, by Medicare—expressed satisfaction. About as many (10%) say it is "the worst possible imaginable system" as say it is the "best possible imaginable system (16%)."[2] Differences were clear along income lines: about two-thirds of people living in households with more than $100,000 of income were happy with U.S. health care, and more than half with incomes hovering near the poverty range ($25,000 to $35,000) were dissatisfied. Many additional studies and surveys—which are designed to assess individual satisfaction with American health care—reach identical conclusions. On the more personal level, a Harris poll in 2000 concluded that many—and perhaps most—people were deeply unhappy with the interaction they had with their own doctors, frustrated that they had to wait for hours for a 5- or 10-minute visit and wondering why they had to take time from their own work just to ask a question or get a referral. Most patients preferred being able to communicate about garden-variety problems or needs via email, and, perhaps unsurprisingly, doctors were often stunned that patients would prefer electronic rather than face-to-face contact.

Taken in the context of a system that is gobbling up an ever greater share of the economy as it grows at a inflation rate three percentage points greater than overall inflation, these large-scale results overwhelm the few—though tangible—successes of modern medicine. Other books address the failings of the health care "system" and provide varying (often mutually contradictory) prescriptions for success. Some advocate greater government oversight,[3] even though most physicians would point to regulations books that are thousands of pages long from Medicare and argue that, despite more rules and restrictions, costs have continued to skyrocket.[4] Market-driven care, they would claim, pushes doctors to chase lucrative insurance contracts with extensive high-tech approaches (almost always paid for by someone other than the actual patients) and beggar much more cost-effective but poorly reimbursed preventative care. Others argue that, as long as employers or government provide health care, there is little incentive for consumers to make choices and force competitive change[5] and that much more in the way of market forces is necessary to bring down the accelerating costs that now tally more than 15% of GDP but leave American's wellness and sense of well-being at best in the middle of the pack among our chief economic competitors in Europe in Asia.

We believe that the current raft of books that examine the American way of doing medicine leave the most important decision makers—people who will one day all be patients—out in the cold. Therefore, in this book, we adopt a very different approach. We focus on providing insights into the management of common chronic diseases of adults, which cause the greatest amount of suffering and which utilize the vast majority of the healthcare budget. There is no question that chronic diseases have the greatest impact on the lives of individuals and the population at large as any with diabetes, heart disease, or cancers of various types knows well.

Our basic philosophy is that, to effect rational change, individuals must—and certainly can—understand the basic medical facts and biology behind the common diseases that account for the vast majority of long-term suffering and the lion's share of health care costs. We endeavor to explain them.

Second, we are convinced that there is overwhelming proof that most—yes, literally most—physicians do not practice medicine based on the scientific evidence readily presented in medical school, required continuing medical education, and medical journals, nor do they pay much attention to the easily available reviews published for free that address dozens of the most common clinical questions physicians face. Thus, well-educated consumers may need to encourage their physicians to gather the latest recommendations or guidelines; it is as we shall show, a bit much to expect physicians to do such analyses themselves both because they are very busy though often with valueless tasks and because they are not trained to do even the simplest statistical analysis of data. We realize that the latter piece of news may be surprising to most readers. We should explain how this unfortunate fact has come about.

Third, many of the common practices in modern medicine, let alone the new and novel, have very few *carefully* done studies to back them up. It is impossible to cover every medical condition and look for so-called "outcome studies" by treatment for all of them. So we discuss the most common problems—the ones each of us is most likely to face—and give the reader enough background and information to ask the right questions, including the hardest one of all: "What happens if I do nothing for a certain condition?" We hope the results will enlighten rather than startle the reader.

Finally, we move beyond concerns for individual health to broader health care policy: how much money are we going to spend? Do we finance health care via taxation? Is universal coverage as desirable a goal as it seems? What is the return on investment? Who pays for research and new treatment trials? Are there more effective and much less costly ways to deliver care for the vast majority of medical needs in the United States? We have constructed the chapters in this book to assist the thoughtful reader in pondering these difficult questions, which will certainly always be debated to some extent and which for the foreseeable future will be a prominent part of the campaigns of each election cycle. While there are no final answers, we believe that the fundamental direction is clear: medical practices should be based in science, and thus any serious policy debate must go beyond how to finance medical care (which is by far the dominant theme and focus in political discourse) to how we make science part of daily medical practice.

As this book attempts to demonstrate, we have a long way to go to realize that goal.

NOTES

1. Available at : http://abcnews.go.com/sections/living/US/healthcare031020_poll .html. Last accessed Nov 9, 2007.
2. Available at: http://health.msn.com/general/zogby_sicko.aspx.
3. Daniel Callhan and Angela A. Wasunna. *Medicine and the Market: Equity vs. Choice* (Baltimore, MD: Johns Hopkins University Press, 2006).
4. James C. Capretta, "What's ailing health care?" *The New Atlantis*, Spring 2007; 16: 69–77.
5. David Gratzer, *The Cure: How Capitalism Can Save American Health Care* (New York: Encounter Press, 2006).

ACKNOWLEDGMENTS

THE AUTHORS would like to acknowledge the editors at AMACOM and, in particular, Associate Editor Mike Sivilli, for hard work done under harder pressure. Every author should be so fortunate to work with a professional who has Mike's sense of humor and near infinite capacity for solving the problems that inevitably crop up in the development and production of a manuscript.

CHAPTER 1

The Medical Prognosis: Why More Is Not Necessarily Better

A dermatologist is someone who knows nothing, and does nothing.
A surgeon is someone who knows nothing, and does everything.
An internist is someone who knows something, and does nothing.
And a pathologist is someone who knows everything, but a day too
late.

> —*Medical field in-joke, author unknown*

LET'S BE UP FRONT with each other from the start: not many people pick up a book on the effectiveness of medical therapies for light reading.

There are readers who are simply health conscious and read books with a medical bent. But most of them are picking up titles on the latest diet. And there are the readers who are doctors, nutritionists, and surgeons by trade who like to read anything related to their passion to heal.

More likely, you're reading this because you or someone close to you is facing a life-changing event—an event that is health related. And one that will force someone to make an irrevocable choice: take chemotherapy, submit to a needle, or go under the tender mercies of the surgeon's knife. It's easy to make a choice about which HMO to go under, which insurance to buy, and even which drug cocktail to imbibe.

But is there really any hard-core information out there that you can use to make that all-important decision: the one that literally could mean life—or the quality of it? We firmly believe that this text is one of the best attempts to give you the edge in these matters. This book is the result of many hours spent researching and reviewing detailed studies on medical applications and patient outcomes.

We have distilled a great deal of information that's difficult for the well-read but nonexpert reader to find outside of the isolated headline in the newspaper. However, if there's one positive development to share in this book, it's that even though the health care system in the United States has its shares of issues, it has carefully acquired years— sometimes even decades—of patient data. And it's this information that tells us the most likely outcomes for a variety of medical problems, particularly for the country's burgeoning population of seniors.

TAKING THE DATA TO HEART

Here's one lesson that the data tells us, over the course of four decades. Before the 1960s, there was little that doctors could do about coronary artery disease. Patients with angina—chest pain from coronary blockages—were simply put to bed rest for several weeks and given aspirin.

It must have seemed like medicine had taken a quantum leap ahead when the cardiac bypass technique was perfected in the later part of the decade. Surgeons would carefully tease out the coronary arteries that supplied blood to the heart muscle as if they were untangling a skein of wool. They would then replace this critical piece of plumbing in a manner similar to doing a pipe repair on an old sprinkler system. Surgeons would carefully remove sections of artery that were clogged with yellowish lumps of congealed fat and replace them with veins harvested from the patient's legs.

Since the veins came from the same patient who was having cholesterol clumps "bypassed," there was no problem with rejection. The rationale for bypass was a simple—and, as it turns out, dramatically oversimplified—belief. It was that blockages in the arteries would lead to angina, the painful constriction or tightness in the chest caused by the depletion of precious oxygen to the heart muscles. If severe enough, the angina might "starve" the heart muscle cells of so much oxygen as to kill those cells: a "heart attack."

The initial successes were splashed across newspaper headlines— and who could blame the media for trumpeting the news? An untreatable condition since it was first described a century prior was suddenly defeatable with the surgeon's knife! With such positive press, it was no surprise that hundreds of thousands of coronary artery bypass grafting procedures (CABG for short—and, yes, it's pronounced "cabbage") were performed each year for the next two decades. At $25,000 per operation or more (in 1984 dollars), this single medical technique out of many hundreds ended up costing the country about 1% or more of its entire health budget at the time.

Shocking? Not nearly as much as the results that the data on patient outcome showed. The truth was that bypass surgery wasn't the cure-all that the medical establishment and the media made it out to be. Simply put, the procedure didn't always work well, and it sometimes resulted in a more rapid demise than if nothing had been done at all!

How could this life-saving therapy have gone wrong? The answer is that in many men, the vein grafts clogged quickly. Worse, because the nerves to the heart that sensed pain were often cut during bypass surgery, patients after the treatment were literally unaware they were still suffering from angina. They simply weren't able to detect the symptoms because the body's wiring had been sheared through and the signals never reached the brain. Billions of dollars were being spent for a procedure that benefited only a fraction of the patients who received it, while arguably harming a great number of the others.

You might next ask, "Why did insurance companies pay for it?" The answer in part is because the surgical procedure became popular from all the good press that surrounded it. In effect, all the free coverage acted like the multitude of drug commercials that we see on television today. Only these endorsements came from the anchor in the newsroom whom you automatically trusted.

It was also in part because the data to show that the surgery was less effective than initially touted would take a lot of time to collect. Obviously, if the surgery resulted in x number of patients expiring on the operating table, the treatment would have been shelved in the nation's medical school libraries next to the studies on snake oil and leeches.

But the results were more subtle than that. It would take years for the data to show that people ended up with unchanged or shorter life spans from bypass surgery. And even the all-knowing odds makers in the insurance companies couldn't access data that didn't exist yet. And just as with the problems that have cropped up with some of the popular medications today, it's a fact that commercially-driven hype moves faster than the slow gathering of data to prove that a treatment actually works.

It's worth asking why a lot of high-technology-based medicine becomes popular. One reason is that the techniques are new; remember, even though bypass surgery has been around a while now, 40 years ago it was perceived as a big jump. Another reason is patients' desperation. And still another, perhaps, is the accolades given to physicians—not to mention the hefty sums paid—for dramatic procedures advertised as "life-saving" and "heroic."

As procedures like bypasses and other high-tech interventions increasingly took over our health care delivery system, the total U.S. health care bill as a percentage of the national gross domestic product ballooned from about 5% in 1980 to over 15% less than 25 years later. That means that health care costs outpaced inflation by factors of 3, 4, and 5 or more over that time; yet life expectancy in the United States lagged profoundly behind Europe, Japan, and Canada where far less was spent per capita on health care.

THE MODERN DOCTOR'S DILEMMA

How could we have ended up in this state? The answers will be explored in this book and will help you talk with your doctor and make better health care choices. In fact, you'll learn the sad truth that the vast majority of physicians are profoundly ill-equipped to know if "doing something" is the same as doing something *useful*.

Don't think that this is yet another book that bashes doctors. We don't think it's necessarily the fault of the medical profession. For the most part, physicians are good people who want to do the best for their patients. But they're like the gamblers going up against the house at a Vegas casino: the system is stacked against them.

In the case of a surprising number of diseases, common sense would seem to dictate that an intervention would, at worst, do no harm. After all, what can be bad about cleaning out a clogged artery? Isn't it the same as cleaning out a clogged drainpipe? But it turns out that the much of what we do in modern American medical practice isn't just worthless and expensive: it's worse than worthless.

And here's a statement that is sure to cause heartburn among some members of the medical profession: the biggest dilemma that doctors face today isn't that they don't have enough options to treat a patient—it's that they have *too many*.

The modern physician has a huge variety of treatment options. You might not think that this is a bad thing; wouldn't you want to have a mechanic work on your car who had a complete set of tools? But here's the catch: most of the "tools" that the doctor uses have *not* been subjected to thorough, scientifically based testing, and biology is so complex that "commonsense" answers are often nonsense.

Furthermore, there are enormous pressures to do something— anything—for an ill patient, even when it's not clear that doing *something* will produce an outcome that is better than doing *nothing*. There are two reasons for this, in our opinion. First, there is more patient pressure to do something than ever before. After all, today's patients are "educated" by the mass media that, whatever their affliction, a little pill will solve the problem. Second, there has been a tremendous increase in the economic benefits to physicians who decide to do something rather than nothing—to do something dramatic to cure a patient instead of taking a more restrained approach.

A DEADLY INTERSECTION: SOFT MEDICINE
AND HARD TECHNOLOGY

After the 1950s the average length of time spent during a visit to the doctor became shorter and shorter. The ultimate cause of this shrinkage is under debate, but during this period, the shift from the family doctor toward today's health maintenance organization (HMO) system started taking place. Whatever the reason, by the 1970s the medical profession seemed to have been won over by the idea that doctors simply didn't spend enough time listening to their patients.

The argument ran pretty much as follows: most visits to the doctor, especially to primary care physicians, are for what are called "functional complaints." These are complaints such as a cold that won't go away, a high fever, an unexplained pain or cramping, and the like. The patient has a symptom or concern that creates understandable anxiety, and, in a vicious circle, the anxiety worsens the symptoms, which increases the anxiety, and so on. Even if the condition wasn't one that could be treated immediately, doing something—anything at all—to decrease the level of anxiety would in turn short-circuit the cycle that was making the patient's symptoms get worse.

The proper way to deal with this kind of problem was to spend more time with the patient—to elicit their concerns. In short, to listen. And, truth be told, it makes sense. (Certainly very few people today would complain that their physicians listen to their complaints too much!)

Medical school admission committees came to an interesting conclusion because of this need to listen to patients. It was felt that people with a liberal arts education would be better able to speak with patients in the way that was needed to properly assess and diagnose complaints. In other words, it would be easier to teach medicine to a good listener than to teach listening skills to a scientifically inclined doctor.

And that was a critical error. If you have to choose between people who are merely scientifically competent and people who are merely socially competent, we believe the correct choice is to choose people with scientific competence. That's simply because the available technology has advanced so far in the past 10 years alone that it is inherently dangerous to use if one doesn't understand the science behind the technology.

Medical school admissions committees began to select individuals who had training in social sciences. And it just so happened that the technological evolution in diagnostics and interventions boomed at the same time. With it a came a sudden, completely unforeseen need for individuals who could wisely choose among a huge number of highly technical choices.

The basic understanding of how equipment or technology works can take time to acquire. More difficult is the practical question of when to use them—and when not! Most people wouldn't expect a doctor to understand how, say, an MRI scanner actually works. But it's essential that the physician understand the limitations of the technology, what it can and cannot show. And there is the ultimate irony of how the two trends—soft medicine and hard technology—came together in a very hazardous way.

We've ended up with a group of physicians who "cared" about their patients but who did not know how to care for them correctly in the scientific sense!

What's the difference between Marcus Welby, MD, and the current generation of physicians? Physicians today have much more opportunity to do harm as well as good. Back in the 1970s, because there was limited availability of technology, there was only so much damage a physician could do. Much of the practice of medicine then was reassurance and recognizing those relatively rare situations where an illness that was not otherwise going to get better on its own (a "self-limited" illness) could be treated with the primitive technology of the day.

UNDERSTANDING THE ODDS CAN EVEN THEM

The ability to practice scientifically correct medicine—which does in fact make a difference in a patient's outcome—depends completely on one's ability to keep up with the medical literature. "Keeping up" means not only reading the literature but actually understanding it. Now most physicians complain that there's simply too much to read.

So we know they aren't reading as much as they should to keep up. But even when they do read, are they understanding what they are reading?

Consider this: one of the keys to understanding how to deploy a new technology or therapy is to understand the odds that it will help or hurt a patient. So doctors need to understand basic statistics. That shouldn't be a problem, right? Doctors are scientifically trained after all, you may think.

Well, not so fast. How much math do you suppose physicians are required to learn? Not as much as you might think! The only absolute requirements for getting into medical school are to take a semester or two of calculus, a freshman physics course, at least one course in basic biology, and at least freshman chemistry and organic chemistry. Beyond that, there are very few additional requirements. In fact, you need a more rigorous background in math to attend graduate business school than to become a surgeon.

Without a solid training in simple statistics at the college level, one cannot read a paper on a new set of treatments and understanding the limitations and risks involved.[1] The question becomes, "Do physicians have the tools to continuously learn and evaluate new techniques and developments throughout their career?" The answer, as we will show, is unequivocally, "No." If physicians cannot critically read scientific papers, they can't determine the right and wrong to do.

THE EVOLUTION OF MEDICAL KNOWLEDGE

Editors of medical journals demand that clinical trials for new treatments or diagnostic approaches be subjected to rigorously controlled scientific scrutiny. The irony is that the vast majority of doctors today who view those studies do not know how to apply the results to patients in their offices. Or, at best, one finds that they can apply the simplest lessons, but not the more complex ones.

Let's take one real-world example. We now know the risk factors that contribute to the likelihood that you'll contract a given disease also affects the outcome of the treatment for those diseases. For example, it was abundantly clear after the Surgeon General's report in the mid- to late 1960s that smoking was strongly associated with lung cancer.

In fact, lung cancer is so strongly associated with smoking that it is extremely rare to have a patient with lung cancer who *hasn't* been a cigarette smoker. So there is effectively a one-to-one, direct, causal relationship between smoking and lung disease. Very few people who smoke on the order of one-half pack or more a day don't develop lung disease of some sort such as emphysema, and very few people who develop lung disease have not smoked. There are exceptions, but they are very rare indeed.[2]

Consequently, the vast majority of scientists and physicians today would say that smoking is not only the major cause of lung cancer; it's also a major cause of noncancerous lung diseases. These would include emphysema or chronic bronchitis, which lead to the need for continuous oxygen therapy and an obviously decreased quality of life.

Now, what if the scenario is a bit more complicated? Let's take the case of a 65-year-old male with advanced heart failure due to atherosclerosis, or hardening of the arteries. In this case, say that it's due (as most cases are) in large measure to decades of heavy smoking.[3] Now that the disease is present, a multitude of risk factors are involved in deciding whether this person is going to benefit from treatment.

If you're the treating physician, it's not hard to come to the correct set of decisions if you know simple statistics. That knowledge allows you to take the data in the literature and assess it for its applicability to your patient's needs by taking his or her history and doing a physical examination. From the history and examination you can learn your patient's risk factors for progression of the disease or for recovery from it based on a given treatment. You would literally be able to calculate the likelihood of success and the likelihood of harm from a given intervention.

The doctor who doesn't know how to evaluate a course of action is using a shotgun approach when a peashooter would work better. To many physicians, the default action is to have a yearly exercise stress test performed on the 65-year-old male patient with established coronary disease.

That sounds prudent, doesn't it? If the stress test is abnormal, then the doctor knows that the patient is at risk for a heart attack. But the physician should have already known that the patient is at risk for a heart attack because he or she has established coronary disease. However, if the stress test is done—and many a cardiologist will do so despite American College of Cardiology recommendations to the contrary—that often leads the physician to order a secondary test to "cover all the bases."

One of the most common secondary tests is a so-called coronary "arteriogram," which has a degree of mortality in and of itself. That is, there's a small but measurable chance that the test itself can kill you! That's because, when you're pushing a plastic catheter into a very narrow artery, you can dislodge deposits of arterial plaque. You can cause the plaque to suddenly flake off and cause a heart attack, or you can find something that, as a cardiologist, you believe needs to be treated.

So you might attempt to put a stent in to widen the narrowed part of the blood vessel to prevent a further heart attack. But there is precious little evidence that a stent makes any difference whatsoever to the long-term survival of the patient. And what makes this an especially poor bargain is that the operation itself makes a tremendous difference to short-term survival; that is, it may kill the patient.

THE DIFFERENCE BETWEEN TRENDS AND INDIVIDUALS

Without an appreciation for the very simplest of statistical analyses, physicians end up using their gut sense or their opinions. Now, once physicians have been in a specialty for 20 or 30 years, for many (and perhaps most) of them, their gut sense is every bit as good as what the statistics tell them. But consider this: the path by which they got to their learned, correct opinion is littered with former patients who have had to live with—or die from—their less than perfect decisions. And, as choices in medical treatments become ever more numerous, complex, and potentially dangerous, it is obvious that better understanding among physicians and other health care providers at the beginning of their careers is essential.

That brings us full circle to why you probably picked up this book: to make sense of the decisions that may be ahead of you or someone you care about, to make decisions based on the hard data, not emotions. You want to make your decisions by the numbers, not by whichever doctor is the smoothest talking or whichever drug company has the best advertisements. And we don't recommend that you use this book as your *only* guide in making your health care decisions. Every person's case is different.

But treat what we have to say as an informed—indeed, as a science-based—"second opinion" when it comes to researching the avenues available. At the very least, it will give you some hard facts to make your decisions, as opposed to the latest commercial for Miracle Drug X on television or the hype to try the latest technical breakthrough in patient care.

During the creation of the book, we also struggled with what statisticians call the "noticeable outliers." That is, we tend to remember the unique or unusual as opposed to the commonplace and average. Indeed, it's only when the man bites the dog that news is made! We can't argue with the fact that, although we might say, "Treatment X hasn't shown any benefit to patients," you might reply, "But I know that Uncle Rob tried X, and it worked."

Treatment X might have indeed worked for your uncle. Or he might have recovered for a reason not connected with the treatment or even in spite of the treatment. All we can point out is that, out of a given sample of people who received a certain treatment, this or that outcome was most common. And when you have an overwhelming number of outcomes that end a certain way, then—to borrow some lingo from Las Vegas—that's betting odds.

NOTES

1. Interestingly enough, basic statistics is a course often required in nursing school, but it is not required in graduate medical school. Very few physicians have ever elected to take a basic statistics course in their undergraduate college years or in medical school. In continuing medical education (CME) courses, which are required for yearly licensure in most states, it is hard to find a single offering in basic statistics.

2. The experience of Dana Reeves notwithstanding, virtually everyone with one of the four common varieties of lung cancer has been or is a heavy cigarette smoker. Yet most of us remember the Dana Reeves story, simply because her life story was both famous and tragic as the wife of actor Christopher Reeve. Indeed, this "recall bias" is a telling characterization of how physicians—like most of us—think based on the most memorable experience, rather than on the entirety of our experience.

3. Yes, we know everyone has a distantly related Uncle Jim who smoked all his life and died at the age of 85 without having even so much as a cough. Because of the natural variation in susceptibility to disease, there is always an exception to the rule. In fact, there cannot not be an "exception" to the rule. But that hardly makes it prudent for anyone to smoke, unless they have reason to believe that their genetic makeup and daily behaviors are otherwise nearly identical to Uncle Jim. Who knew that Uncle Jim spent eight hours a day chopping down trees and dragging them out of the forest, ate wild (antioxidant-containing) berries for breakfast and lunch, and was a vegetarian at dinnertime?

C H A P T E R 2

Dissecting the Practice of Medicine

MORE THAN 40 YEARS AGO, a professor named Dan Wennberg at the Dartmouth Medical School began a study that would, for the first time, begin to "quantify" the way medicine is practiced in the United States. In the years following World War II, the number of physicians grew tremendously, but most of the specialties of medicine were in their early stages of development. For the most part, physicians were generalists, taking care of all age groups, though some "hospital-based" specialties, such as radiology and anesthesiology, were attracting increasing numbers of medical school graduates. At about the time that these hospital-based specialists began to install and utilize new equipment—X-ray machines of various types that could do more than just imagine broken bones or the lungs, anesthesia equipment for the precise delivery of potentially dangerous medications during surgery—more aggressive and previously unthinkable surgical procedures were working their way into medical practice. Vascular surgery, heart valve operations, and even delicate procedures to remove tumors of the brain and the spinal cord, which simply were not previously possible, became routine. Medicine was entering a technological boom in the 1960s, one that has continued to this day, leading to ever more complex procedures, in turn necessitating highly specialized training for the physicians who apply these techniques.

Professor Wennberg noticed that as new procedures became available and clearly described in the medical literature, the *indications* for those procedures were often ambiguous. In other words, physicians were trying new approaches for a multiplicity of previously untreatable diseases, but, because the diseases were generally rare, few physicians or even large institutions would have dozens of cases and outcomes that could be published and reviewed by other physicians. Thus, from place to place within cities and across states, there was enormous variation in the use of the new technologies and surgical techniques that were erupting in medicine. Unsurprisingly, not only did physicians' training and experience vary, but so did the patients themselves—by age, gender, general physical health, education, socioeconomic status—all characteristics that we now know dramatically affect outcomes even when a specific procedure or medication is used to treat a specific disease. Thus Wennberg realized that a "natural experiment" was taking place: dozens of new diagnostic machines for identifying ever more complex diseases and multiple novel surgical approaches for treating those diseases meant that some patients would receive new therapies, some older therapies, and some none at all based mostly on the whim or training of the physician. He was interested not only in the outcomes of the different approaches, but also in how frequently the new technologies or techniques were used. In other words, he wanted to know how much variation there was in the practice of physicians for various conditions, what scientists usually refer to as "statistical variance."

Now, you might think that variability in treating conditions is to be expected. But Wennberg wasn't studying a cross-section of people throughout society. He was looking at what was supposed to be one of the most highly trained—and highly standardized—set of professional people around: medical doctors. Given that many new procedures were rapidly entering the repertoire of practitioners, one would have assumed that from the very introduction of these practices a careful analysis of outcomes would be published so as to know how many patients or even what kinds of patients—based on age, gender, and other criteria—were being helped and who might actually be made worse off. Just because a new procedure seems to make sense doesn't mean that it always does good. Wennberg realized that no organized, comprehensive analysis of the plethora of new methods and diagnostic tests was required of physicians and that few were undertaking such an analysis on their own initiative. It was particularly striking that in all other scientific and engineering fields this kind of analysis was routine. Yet, in medicine where individual's lives were directly at stake, it wasn't happening. There was no way to know—aside from individual case reports published in scattered medical journals—if the new "breakthroughs" in medicine were making a positive difference, made no difference, or perhaps even caused worse outcomes. As we shall see, even to this day, the same problem exists with the introduction of new medicines or technologies. What is clear is that **costs** *have skyrocketed, but benefits are much harder to show.*

So consider this analogy. Imagine that you are in an elevator in a public building in downtown Los Angeles. You're just coming down from the twentieth floor with a dozen other passengers when an earthquake hits. No one is physically injured, but the power goes out, the cable goes loose, and the emergency brakes kick in before the car falls. You learn via cell phone that, due to the magnitude of the quake, no one is likely to come for at least a couple hours, and you smell smoke.

That's a *very* stressful situation. You might think—and you'd be correct—that a random sampling of people who happen to be on the elevator with you would all think and react differently. Some might panic, others might argue to stay put, and others would try to pry a way out or call for help. Since no one on the elevator is likely to be professionally trained in what to do in this situation, the variation in reactions among the trapped people would be great.

Now suppose that the same earthquake takes place, you're stranded on the elevator, but you happen to be in the company of 11 trained, veteran firefighters. That's unlikely, of course, but let's say that they're in town for the annual Ladder n' Hose Expo. Would you get the same degree of variability in their reactions? Almost certainly not. And the difference between the two scenarios is the level of training and knowledge—the exact thing that would, in theory, set doctors apart when it came to handling unfamiliar cases.

THE NO-SUM GAME

The Dartmouth study on variations in medical practice reviews the Medicare database, collected by the Health Care Finance Administration, a quasi-independent branch of the federal government. The study—which continues as of the writing of this book—has been designed to answer three questions of importance to patients, physicians, health care planners, and even insurance companies in their attempt to determine how much to pay for various physician services as well as to estimate the future health care costs of the Medicare population. These questions are:

- For the most commonly done—and often very expensive— medical procedures in the Medicare population, after taking into account the severity of a given illness, the presence of other complicating medical conditions, and the age, gender, and race of a patients in the population, how likely is it that a given medical procedure will be used for a certain medical condition in different communities?

- If there are differences in the use of certain procedures or differences in physician decision making, what is the difference in outcome for a given medical problem? "Outcome" is measured in both the quality of life and the quantity of addition life, and there are well accepted methods for quantifying these outcomes.

- Finally, what factors are most likely to account for the variation in the use of medical procedures, including surgical interventions and radiology studies (e.g., MRI scans, CT scans, and the like)? Does it have to do with the number of physicians, the training of physicians, their age, or their location in the United States?

It is important to point out that Wennberg and his colleagues used Medicare data because it is the only, more or less complete database on the medical care delivered (or actually "billed") to a portion of the U.S. population. Most members of that population, of course, are elderly, although there are some people under the age of 65 who receive Medicare as well. No similar data exists in any one place for the under-65 population because it is owned by insurance companies and health maintenance organizations, considered "proprietary," and thus never published. Since the federal government pays for just about all Medicare expenditures, it can make its data publicly known (stripped of specific patient identifiers to protect patient confidentiality).

Equally important to understand is that, for the most part, Wennberg looked at outcomes toward the end of life—roughly the last year or so of life—for most of his analysis. The reason for doing so was to identify those members of the population who are truly ill (for, after all, most of the patients died within 6 to 12 months of a particular procedure or medical intervention being performed). This eliminates much variability in severity of disease, per se; it is hard to argue that many of the patients were in robust health to start off with, thus decreasing the chance that any variability in the use of medical procedures could be ascribed to the severity of illness in individuals.

Because most of the medical interventions Wennberg studied are expensive (e.g., a coronary bypass operation can easily cost in excess of $40,000 when hospital and physician charges are taken into account), one simple way to address the question of variability is to look at total Medicare expenditure in the last few months of life. In turn, one way to look at expenditure is in terms of the total number of hospital days that terminally ill Medicare recipients spend in the hospital across the roughly 300 areas of the country that Medicare indicates as hospital referral regions (HRRs). By "terminally ill," the Dartmouth researchers meant only people who would go on to die within six months of a hospital admission.

In Figure 2-1, each dot represents one hospital region (thus there are 306 dots in total in the U.S.), and on the vertical axis is plotted the number of days spent in hospital sometime during the last six months of life. The results are astounding—but reproduced for a wide variety of other measurements of variation in services in the Medicare population. Depending on what part of the country one lives in, during the last half year of life, one can expect to spend somewhere between 5 and 20 days in the hospital—a variation of a factor of 4.

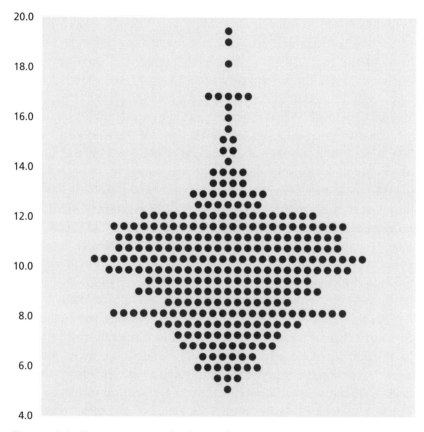

FIGURE 2-1. Patient days in the hospital during the last six months of life among medicare decedents in 306 hospital referral regions (2003). [From *A Dartmouth Atlas Project Topic Brief: Supply-Sensitive Care* (Hanover, NH: Dartmouth College, Center for the Evaluative Clinical Sciences, November 14, 2005), available at www.dartmouthatlast.org].

4237796

You might be thinking that some variation would be expected. For example, it is true that some sections of the country are poorer than others and that individuals' levels of wellness and access to preventive service can therefore be expected to vary, perhaps resulting in some variation for terminal care. But is it reasonable that, across the United States, a three- to four-fold variation in necessary hospital days would result based on these explanations? Could something else be driving these huge differences across the country?

It is impossible to prove that such is *not* the case—just as proving any negative statement or "ruling out" a possibility is very difficult. But it is possible to make a given explanation less credible by offering other hypotheses and supporting information. In this case, the Dartmouth group believes that, while there might be some variance in the number of hospital days used by patients who are soon to die because of differences in disease or accident patterns, in the underlying socio-economic status, and in the education of patients and other factors, a more credible explanation is that the variation is driven by physicians and hospitals themselves.

How might one test such a theory? Consider the following. For a few conditions there is, for all intents and purposes, no choice in what kind of care or treatment is selected, whereas for other conditions there might be a wide variety of choices for treatment. In the former category there is a classic example: a hip fracture.

If one is unfortunate enough to fall and break the top of the femur (the "thigh" bone) near where it joins the pelvis at the hip, surgery is required (almost always involving replacement of a portion of the femur or putting the pieces of the femur back together). Indeed, before such surgical options were available, many people would languish in pain for weeks or months—and often go on to die from this problem. Today, hip replacement surgery is universally available and safe, and it almost always gives a good result (thanks mostly to advances in engineering materials to replace the broken portion of the femur and better anesthesia methods, permitting sometimes lengthy surgery to be undertaken safely and having little to do with the orthopedist's skills). Thus, one would expect that most people who have a hip fracture get hip replacement surgery, and, as we'll see momentarily, indeed they do.

It is possible to compare the rate of hip replacement surgery and the rate of hospitalization for other conditions with each other and with a possible hidden driver for hospitalizations, for example the number of hospital beds or physicians in a community. If the variation in health care intensity in the United States is, in fact, widespread due to factors *other* than medically justifiable reasons (such as physician preference or the desire of hospital administrators to keep their beds full and earning income), then we would expect to see a strong correlation between "elective" admissions and, say, hospital beds in the community but no such correlation between the rate of admissions for hip replacement and acute hospital beds. In the latter, there is simply no choice. The patient must be admitted for surgery and rather extensive postoperative care.

And that is precisely what the Dartmouth group found, as Figure 2-2 shows. On the vertical axis is plotted the number of hospital discharges per 100,000 individuals in one of the 306 HRRs, and on the horizontal axis is the number of acute care hospital beds per 1,000 people in those same regions. No matter how many hospital beds are available, the discharges (or admissions) for patients with a hip fracture is the same in every part of the country. But for all other medical problems—where there is almost always a judgment involved in whether an admission is truly necessary—there is a close relationship between the number of hospital beds available and the total number of admissions in any given year. The correlations are very strong; more than 50% (54% to be precise) of the variation in hospital admission rates across the country for a wide variety of medical conditions is explained—at least from the statistical standpoint—by how much space is available to admit patients in the first place.

Generally, hospital admissions are, of course, very expensive, and if patients are being admitted unnecessarily (as would almost certainly seem to be the case), then many hundreds of billions of dollars are being spent without good reason. Even worse, as we shall see shortly, there is no evidence that, in areas that are better supplied with hospital beds and that in turn admit more patients per capita, the outcomes from treating conditions as inpatients—or "intensively"—as opposed to as outpatients is any better. In fact, there is ever more compelling

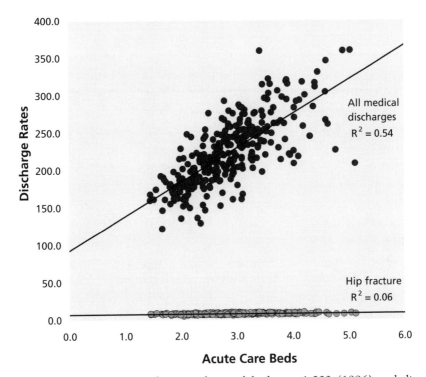

FIGURE 2-2. Association between hospital beds per 1,000 (1996) and discharges per 1,000 (1995–1996) among Medicare enrollees in 306 hospital referral regions.

evidence that the outcome is *worse* the more intensive the treatment is, even when one takes into account how serious disease in given individuals happens to be.

You might argue that higher hospital admission rates occur in areas where there are more hospitals because patients are sent from areas where there are fewer beds. But close examination of detailed data shows that this explanation doesn't hold either. It seems unavoidable that something other than necessary treatment is being delivered and on a very, very large scale across the entire country.

Another piece of evidence that undermines the notion that some geographic or patient-related variable could account for the contrasting rates of hospital admissions is seen in Figure 2-3.[1] In this case, the Dartmouth researchers tested the hypothesis that using an orthopedic

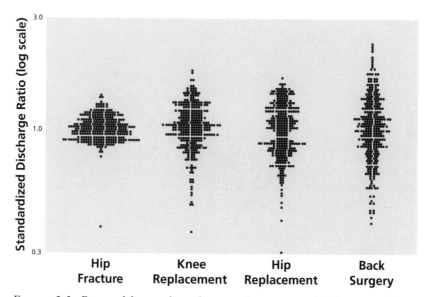

FIGURE 2-3. Rates of four orthopedic procedures among Medicare enrollees in 306 hospital referral regions (2002–2003).

procedure (hip replacement) as a basis for comparison with all other medical procedures might be unfair—that is, something unique about orthopedic practice differentiates it from the rest of medicine. Yet that too turns out not to be the case. When hip replacement in the setting of *hip fracture*—an unavoidable choice on the part of the doctor and patient—is compared to *elective* orthopedic procedures—knee replacement for osteoarthritis, hip replacement for osteoarthritis, and back surgery (usually for chronic pain or degenerative changes in the disks of the back)—another staggering result emerges. For elective orthopedic procedures (where nothing is forcing the use of invasive and expensive operations, save for rare cases), variations are extreme across the country.[2] Especially for back operations—almost always based on the opinion of an orthopedic surgeon as opposed to being dictated by near absolute necessity, as in the case of operations for hip fracture—variations are extreme, more than seven times as great as when surgeons are considering what to do for hip fracture patients.

In Figure 2-3, each dot represents a single HRR (there are thus 306 dots for each of the four operations). Thus, another way to easily understand this graph is as follows: given that the "average" rate for an operation is defined to be 1, if all the dots cluster near 1, there isn't much variation. If, however, the dots are spread out dramatically in the vertical direction, there is a great deal of variation in the use of orthopedic procedures for each condition.

As expected, the rate of hip fracture surgeries is about the same across the country—almost all of the dots are near 1 on the vertical axis of the graph. Also, hip fracture surgery rates may be a bit less or more than 1. This could be due to the fact that some patients die before receiving surgery, or that some patients require more than one operation to correct their hip fractures.

But look instead at the other three orthopedic procedures: the variation in the use of back surgery (almost always for degenerative arthritis of the back, as is common in older people) varies by a factor of about 10 across the country; for hip replacement (for degenerative arthritis, not fracture), the variation is about a factor of 5; and for knee replacement (again almost always for degenerative arthritis), the factor is 4. Given the costs of these three procedures—easily $10,000 and $20,000 in most locations in the country—the amount of money spent per Medicare recipient for these operations fluctuates enormously across the United States.

As the authors of the Dartmouth Atlas themselves comment on the information in Figure 2-3:

> In theory, the differences among these communities in rates of knee and hip replacement and about treatment, or the incidence of osteoarthritis and/or herniated discs. In light of the evidence, this seems unlikely. Moreover, there is no epidemiologic evidence that illness or informed patient preferences vary as sharply according to the boundaries of health care markets as does surgery. It seems very unlikely that differences in illness rates and/or patient preferences could account for rates of knee, hip and back surgery.

As we'll see in detail in Chapter 3, there is no difference in outcome as more money is spent (in fact, even worse, outcomes often get worse as more money is spent). We can get a taste for this unpleasant result by considering the following situation addressed by the Dartmouth group: if we look at three common conditions in the Medicare population as a whole—hip fracture, colon cancer, and heart disease—and divide the amount spent into five groups from highest expenditure per patient to lowest expenditure per patient and then compare outcomes of the highest quintile (called "Q5") of expenditure with the lowest quintile (called "Q1"), the results for cost are as follows:

Resource Inputs

Resource	Ratio, Q5 vs. Q1
Per-capita Medicare spending	1.61
Hospital beds per 1,000	1.32

In other words, the "most expensive" group is 1.6 times as expensive as the least expensive group with exactly the same condition.

The results for outcome are shown in the next table:

Cohort Health Outcomes

Condition	Relative risk of death, Q5 vs. Q1	95% CL
Hip fracture	1.019	(1.0007–1.0386)
Colon cancer	1.052	(1.0123–1.0936)
Heart attack	1.052	(1.0177–1.0884)

In other words, the risk of death from the procedure is higher—by as much as 5%—in the most expensive group as the least expensive group.

Finally, when patients were examined and interviewed a few months after their procedure, they described their functional status—their ability to walk or carry out the activities of daily living—as the same in the high expenditure group vs. the low expenditure group. Their satisfaction level was no different except on one measure: patients in the highest expenditure group thought that their "access to care" was **worse** *than those in the lowest expenditure group.*

Now you may be thinking that perhaps the high expenditure group had a worse outcome—that is, a higher risk of death—because they were somehow sicker or more frail. But that is not the explanation because all of those considerations were taken into account in the Dartmouth analysis. To put it another way, something other than severity of illness (or age, gender, education, or socioeconomic status) accounted for the variation in *both* the actual use of procedures and the adverse results from the use of those procedures.

As a result of the tremendous variation in the use of almost any expensive modern surgical procedure across the United States, facts such as these emerge:

- A typical 65-year-old in Miami will cost Medicare $50,000 more in his or her lifetime than a 65-year-old in Minneapolis, enough to pay for a Lexus with all the trimmings.

- Three of every 1,000 Medicare beneficiaries undergo heart bypass surgery each year in Albuquerque, but 11 per 1,000 do in Redding, California.

- Only 14% of the terminally ill in Sun City, Arizona, enter an intensive care unit in the last six months of life, but 49% do in Sun City, California.

- Elderly men in Binghamton, New York, are nine times more likely to have their prostate removed than men of the same age in Baton Rouge.

We'll explore more information on variations in cardiac, urologic, and orthopedic care in the next chapter. We will also look at the consequences—almost all of them adverse—as a result of focusing far too much on high-technology, expensive care, while forgetting to do the simple (and less well reimbursed) things that make the biggest difference in outcome for patients with the most common of diseases, the ones that cause the greatest loss of life in the United States.

THE VALUE YOU'RE GETTING

At this point, most readers probably are asking the natural questions: "What explains this variance in the use of all of these expensive—and obviously dangerous—procedures? Is our money spent for good reason?"

Because the Dartmouth study is "retrospective"—that is, it looks at events after they happen—as any statistician will tell you, there is no good way to know for certain what factors account for the profound variance. However, we can postulate explanations—"reasonable" on their face to most people—to see if those factors are correlated with the variance in medical expenditures. Bear in mind that statistical correlation is not the same as causation. But if the explanatory factors are plausibly connected to the outcome, then we may have a better understanding not only of why health care costs vary so much across the United States, but also of what to do about it.

Let's start with the doctors themselves. Perhaps, as is the case with the number of lawyers in a community, where one would expect that the number and length of lawsuits are related to the number of attorneys per capita, it may be the case that if there are lots of doctors around to do things, then more money would be spent on medical procedures. After all, it's doctors who drive admissions to the hospital and who order laboratory tests, the number of X-rays ordered, and procedures or consultations with other physicians. In fact, *only physicians and physician assistants can do these things. As we see from the results of the Dartmouth analysis in Figure 2-4, the more physicians there are per capita, the higher the costs are.*

About three-quarters of all the variance in total expenditure that we saw in the previous graphs can be explained by how many services physicians deliver. Put another way, the more physicians there are involved in a given case, the greater the costs are. That's not necessarily a surprise because it may be the case that sicker patients simply need more physicians; so the cost increase per patient would be fine if those physicians in the upper right-hand corner of Figure 2-4 got a better result than those who were in the lower left-hand corner. Unfortunately, they don't.

Many examples illustrate this regrettable result; let's look at a representative one.

It is now very well established that people who have suffered a heart attack (and survive; perhaps 30% to 40% of people with heart

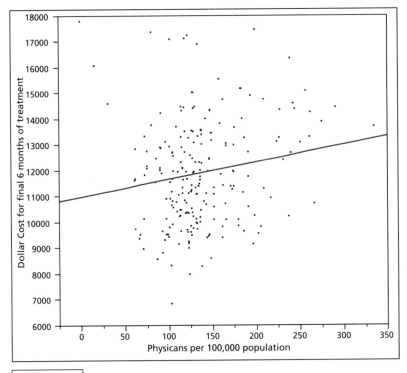

— Linear Fit

Linear Fit
Dollar Cost for final 6 months of treatment = 10970.833 + 6.7330035 Physicans per 100,000 population

Summary of Fit

RSquare	0.026429
RSquare Adj	0.022004
Root Mean Square Error	2006.822
Mean of Response	11893.52
Observations (or Sum Wgts)	222

Analysis of Variance

Source	DF	Sum of Squares	Mean Square	F Ratio
Model	1	24052147	24052147	5.9722
Error	220	886013265	4027333	**Prob > F**
C. Total	221	910065412		0.0153

Parameter Estimates

Term	Estimate	Std Error	t Ratio	Prob>|t|
Intercept	10970.833	400.8634	27.37	<.0001
Physicans per 100,000 population	6.7330035	2.755121	2.44	0.0153

Figure 2-4. Costs per person as physicians' numbers rise in a community.

attacks die immediately or shortly after being taken to the hospital) will have much better quality of life as well as a longer life if they receive a certain class of heart medication called "angiotensin converting enzyme inhibitors," or "ACE inhibitors" for short. ACE inhibitors are inexpensive and convenient to take, only on rare occasions do they have any serious side effects, and their benefits are unequivocally large. So one would expect that the more doctors that get involved—and the greater the intensity of services provided to a heart attack victim—the greater the likelihood that the patient would walk out of the hospital with a prescription for an ACE inhibitor, right? It turns out that exactly the opposite is true, as is shown in Figure 2-5.

Each point in this graph represents a single area of the country and the patients are more-or-less the same: they've suffered a heart attack and survived to walk out of the hospital. But oddly, the more doctors involved, the less likely the patient is to get the correct pre-

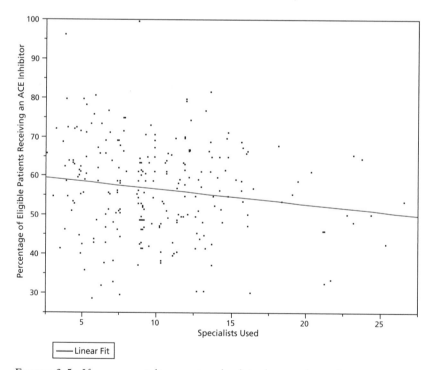

FIGURE 2-5. If more specialists are involved, is the care better?

scription for an ACE inhibitor. Overall the likelihood itself—from about 30% to 85 or 90%—is worrisome. But even more troubling is that as a general rule (indicated by the red "trend line" in the graph), the more doctors involved, the worse the "quality" of care, in this case measured by the failure to prescribe an effective, inexpensive medicine to heart attack patients. Similar results are found for other very simple, effective interventions as we will detail later in this book.

Of course, just because two factors happen coincidentally, you cannot assume causation. As we noted earlier, it is always important to ask, "Are there other explanations?" For example, is there some other way to explain the variation in the treatment of patients with a very well studied, extremely common problem when we are *certain* of the benefits from those simple interventions? Despite years of trying, there is no valid scientific explanation save for this: the medical system fails as more and more doctors get involved. Perhaps the problem is a lack of communication. Perhaps there are so many doctors that there is no captain of the ship, so the simple things get overlooked as each specialist focuses on his or her narrow area of expertise; perhaps the explanation is akin to missing the forest because trees are blocking the view.

And, as it turns out, the same conclusion applies for patients with orthopedic problems, cancers, and even generally minor problems who would otherwise be expected to live for a long time: more care results in neither longer lifespan, better quality of life, nor quicker recovery from acute mild illnesses.

For end-of-life care, we have an especially clear-cut example of the lack of efficacy of more intensive treatment. Given the enormous variation in dollars spent in the last six months of life for the average Medicare patient, it is difficult to conclude that variation in the severity of illness explains the variation in intensity of care, simply because everyone in this group is clearly very ill. In other words, we're limiting the possibility in a lot of variation in the patient's condition because they are all in similar situations—suffering from a combination of acute and chronic conditions that plague many of us at the end of our lifespan. Therefore, if interventions made any difference, we'd expect to see them in the outcomes of these patients—a longer (though obviously limited) life span or better quality of life. The data does not support this conclusion. In fact, from the Dartmouth study, excessive care leads to an increased relative risk of mortality of about 3% as shown in Figure 2-6.

PAINTING BY NUMBERS

As is probably now clear, the Dartmouth study is an attempt to *quantify* and then to try to *understand* medical reasoning, specifically, to identify the root cause or causes for the profound variation in the use of a variety of common physician and hospital services across the country for given conditions. And after many years of research, the Dartmouth Group, which is trying to influence health care policy as well as reduce spiraling medical costs has come up with three major conclusions.

The first conclusion of the Dartmouth study is that, just like the variation in overall care for a given medical condition, there is an equal variation in the use of those few treatments recognized to be

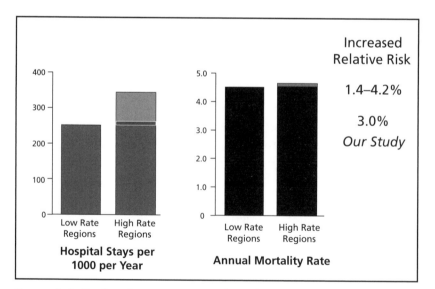

FIGURE 2-6. Predicted impact on mortality of excess supply-sensitive hospitalizations.

truly effective. "Effective" care means care for which there is evidence that it positively affects both the quality and quantity of life that a patient receives.

FLIPPING A COIN ON A HEART ATTACK

Let's continue with the observation that has been made and reproduced in multiple widely read medical journals on the variation in the use of effective care. An excellent example is heart disease. Beta blockers are an inexpensive medication that are known to reduce the recurrence of heart attacks in people who have already had them.

Beta blockers were developed in the 1950s and 1960s by Dr. Eugene Braunwald, the famous Harvard cardiologist, and they were originally used for the treatment of high blood pressure. But it was observed that patients who had had a heart attack, for which obviously high blood pressure is one of the most common risk factors, seemed to do better in the long term if the blood pressure was controlled with a particular class of medications (hypertensive medications) than with other medications.

It was observed that beta blockers, which slow down the heart rate a bit by decreasing the force with which the heart contracts, may also affect blood circulation. It does this by enlarging blood vessels all over the body but, for all intents and purposes, they appear to work mostly by interfering with adrenalin or one of its close cousins called norepinephrine.[3]

This conferred a survival advantage for patients who received beta blockers instead of other medications that lower their blood pressure to an equivalent extent. So there was something about beta blockers that went beyond their efficacy in lowering blood pressure. Thus, it helped in preventing—not absolutely but to a very large degree—a second coronary event.

In the 1980s, a set of trials was done across the country in which patients with known coronary disease who generally had a high risk for heart attacks were divided into groups. One group received beta blockers, while a second received diuretic medication. The third received what was then a very popular class of drugs (popular with the pharmaceutical industry because they were new and expensive), called calcium channel blockers.

All these medications reduced blood pressure equivalently. But it became abundantly clear that patients who received beta blockers did better than either of the other two groups. Startlingly, those who received the new and expensive calcium channel blockers actually did worse than those who received either the beta blockers or diuretics. Diuretics were the oldest of all high blood pressure medications. The diuretics which were, by far, the cheapest medications, were more effective than the extremely expensive calcium channel blockers. And the beta blockers were the most effective of all, even though they were a little more expensive than the diuretics.

So the use of beta blockers became a quality measure that is followed by Medicare, HMOs, and even the Dartmouth Group to see just what percentage of people across the country who have had a heart attack leave the hospital with a prescription for a beta blocker in hand. Based on effectiveness, just about everyone should leave the hospital with such a prescription, but it turns out that only about 45% of heart attack patients do.

One of the additional striking finds of the study was that there was no difference between academic medical centers, where you would think that the best care would be provided, compared to local hospitals that were not necessarily associated with medical schools. That's terrible! Here we have a very inexpensive medication that is *proven* to reduce the risk of recurrence of heart attacks, the need for hospitalization, and the risk of heart failure. Yet less than half the time do academic physicians—cardiologists included—make sure that their patients receive it.[4]

Physicians seem to make sure that the expensive procedures are done (because they are lucrative), but they don't take care of the "little" things that turn out to be at least as important as the expensive interventions. Despite their tarnished reputation with much of the public, large HMOs have been best able to control and fix this problem. That's because HMOs like Kaiser Permanente, for instance, make it a matter of policy to ensure that all of their heart attack patients—

unless they have some contraindication for the medication—get their beta blockers.

The situation gets even worse when you consider that there is an even simpler medication for preventing a second heart attack and, indeed, for preventing a first heart attack: plain old aspirin tablets. Aspirin has been shown in countless studies to be extraordinarily effective in preventing a second heart attack, assuming that we don't have a stomach ulcer or some other reason that you can't take aspirin.

Yet, across the country on average, only about 60% of patients with heart attacks walk out of the hospital and have been instructed to take a baby aspirin a day. These two inexpensive medications together, a beta blocker and aspirin, perhaps cost on the order of 25¢ to 50¢ per day, but they reduce the risk of death overall in patients with heart disease by more than 20% in any given year. Over the course of several years, the cumulative reduction in death rate just from taking aspirin is much greater—perhaps nearly 40% or 50% in patients who continue taking this old but very potent medication. And, when the total number of heart attack victims every year is taken into account, the number of years of extra life lived—most of it with good quality and functioning—is enormous.

A STROKE IN THE EYE

So the first conclusion of the Dartmouth Study was pretty startling. Even when there is a known, inexpensive, effective medical intervention—the use of beta blockers and aspirin after heart attacks—there's no better chance than a flip of a coin that you'll be given the correct prophylactic medication when you leave the hospital.

The story is the same for many other common diseases. The best examples of these are diabetes and high blood pressure.

One of the most troublesome problems that diabetics face is that they develop blockages in the tiny blood vessels of the retina of the eye (the retina is the surface at the back of the eyeball). When these little blood vessels develop blockages, the tissue surrounding them in the retina, of course, dies, because the cells require large amounts of energy and oxygen because they are very active. Think about it; at any time day or night we have come to expect that when are eyes are open or opened after sleeping, the retinal cells immediately spring into action, literally within a fraction of a second. Such responsiveness, not to mention the function of turning light into images that your brain can interpret and act upon, requires large quantities of nutrients on an absolutely continuous basis. Should that supply be cut off, even for a few seconds or a minute, the metabolically active cells use up their limited stores of energy-rich molecules and the very machinery inside the cell that maintains their delicate and profoundly powerful structure begins to collapse. The cell becomes, in the words of the pathologist, "necrotic," and undergoes an irreversible process, only recently described and not well understood, called "apoptosis"—programmed cell death. Just as in the rest of the brain (for the eye is anatomically and functionally part of the brain), this cell death is a "stroke"—a sudden onset of dysfunction in the back of the eyeball.

Then, on the border of the dead cells, other cells are barely getting enough of a blood supply. And what they do is to exude a hormone-like substance that stimulates the growth of new blood vessels so that they can get more oxygen and other nutrients in order to survive. In scientific terms, the process is called "neovascularization."

Now that sounds good, except that the hormone-like substance the cells exude is so powerful it causes a very rich growth of new blood vessels in the area. These new vessels are extremely fragile and extremely numerous—almost like an unwieldy growing tangle of tiny vessels with shoddy foundations—and so they tend to bleed.

As a result of bleeding in the retina, the cells of the retina literally get lifted off the surface. That causes a retinal detachment, which leads to a loss of vision not in just a small portion of the visual field but in a large portion of it. We now have known for more than a decade that, if one detects the presence of these small, new proliferative blood vessels, something can be done. We can zap the vessels with a laser before they can either bleed or exude more of the hormone that causes more blood vessel growth. In this manner, we can almost completely prevent retina detachment from hemorrhage, which is the single largest cause of blindness among diabetics.

And so Medicare recommends that diabetics have yearly eye examinations done, preferably by an optometrist or ophthalmologist. This is because these specialists have the special optical equipment to be able to see out to the periphery of the retina, whereas the doctor with a standard ophthalmoscope can see only a portion of it. If these proliferative blood vessels are found, you can reduce the probability of blindness tremendously, perhaps by a factor of four or five, by killing off those new, abnormal blood vessels with a laser. In other words, neovascularization is an "inappropriate" response to retinal cell death in that it creates a situation where further retinal damage is almost certain to occur; it's as if the body's repair mechanism for the damage diabetes does in the eye wasn't designed to deal with the problem correctly. Thus, by stopping the neovascularization—literally by destroying the new blood vessels with a laser as well as some of the cells that are pouring out growth factors that create these fragile, dysfunctional blood vessels—further visual loss can be stopped. We should note that visual loss that has already occurred cannot, in general, be recovered by this process, but at least we can prevent what would otherwise be a downward spiral into nearly complete destruction of vision.

Yet, in 2001, less than half of all Medicare enrollees with diabetes had a yearly eye examination. In the very, very best regions, the number was as high as 75%, but in no region did it get anywhere near 100%. That finding was consistent as well for academic medical centers, including famous ones such as the Mayo Clinic, Stanford University, University of Chicago, and Harvard Medical School.

There was no difference either within the academic medical centers themselves; with rare exceptions, one outpatient clinic of an academic medical center system did about as well (or as poorly) as another outpatient center.

UNDER PRESSURE

Another important disease to reflect upon is high blood pressure and the failure of effective care in this common disorder. High blood pressure affects roughly more than a third (and some studies suggest up to

40%) of Americans at some time in their life, obviously more in the older age groups. The algorithms and guidelines for choosing appropriate blood pressure medications have been developed over the course of about the past 30 years and continuously refined and updated on almost a yearly basis and published in journals, such as the *Journal of the American Medical Association* (JAMA), the single most widely read journal in all of medicine.

But if one studies people with high blood pressure, based on the most recently published data, about two-thirds of patients did not receive the recommended care (and many received no care at all). Either the care was inadequate, the most cost-effective medications were somehow overlooked, or the blood pressure elevations weren't treated at all. The reason for treating high blood pressure isn't to make the numbers look good, but rather, that people with high blood pressure face a much increased risk of heart attack, stroke, and death, *and* we also know that those risks can be largely mitigated by keeping blood pressure under control.

Thus, the most striking conclusion of the Dartmouth study to date is that, even for those very few things that physicians do that we *know* are effective, the medical community has failed to do them correctly. It's not hard to tell heart attack survivors to take a baby aspirin and to write a prescription for a beta blocker, nor is it expensive and unaffordable for the overwhelming majority of people. Similarly, for the extraordinarily common problem of blood pressure, treatment can be had for far less than a dollar a day in the vast majority of patients.

For the older population group, Medicare covers those expenses completely. Something is terribly wrong when the simple things that make the most difference are missed, especially when paying for them isn't a problem.

BEYOND MEDICARE

The Dartmouth study gives some tantalizing hints that the problem isn't limited to the Medicare population. The reason is this: in just about every medical specialty one examines, the same variations in the delivery of services seen already among orthopedic surgeons can be found. Wennberg and colleagues have looked at urology, cardiology, radiology, and general surgical procedures, and the finding is the same. Consider Figure 2-7, which summarizes the rate of use of a wide variety of expensive medical procedures in the 300-odd hospital reporting regions in the United States.

As before, the clever user of a "control" group—patients with hip fractures who almost always require a repair (there simply isn't much leeway in what do to for these patients)—allows a comparison. Each Rorschach-like blotch of frequency of use of procedures tells the same story. In fact, the *less* evidence there is for the actual life-saving or life-improving value of a procedure, the *greater* the variability.

IS IT AS BAD AMONG YOUNGER POPULATIONS?

Some people in the health care community might be skeptical about the results of the Dartmouth study, extensive as it is and as consistent as the conclusions seem to be. They will assert that in younger age

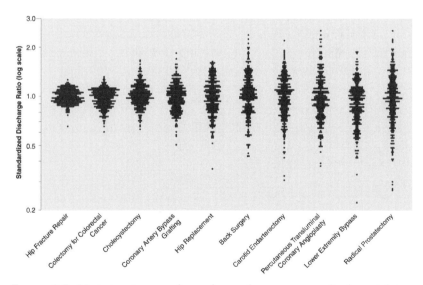

FIGURE 2-7. Variation in rate of use of procedures across medical specialties.

groups, medical care is better, and they might further argue that, since older people have so many problems per person, any attempt to look at a disease in isolation—despite the statistical adjustments so painstakingly made by the Dartmouth researchers—is just nonsense, not the basis for changes in public policy. Are they right?

Until very recently, it was impossible to answer this question because, unlike the Medicare population, there is no central database of health care outcomes that is accessible to researchers. Most HMOs, clinics, and individual physicians' offices don't make a practice of publishing their results for competitors to see. The very limited data available was restricted to a few diseases, to small geographic areas, or to relatively poor children covered by the Medicaid program. The available information was simply not representative of children across the country, and thus an entire new set of studies—expensive and hard to do—were necessary.

One such study has just been published in the prestigious *New England Journal of Medicine.*[5] The news is shocking, even when the possible limitations of the authors' work is taken into account. When the medical records of over 1,500 children in 12 metropolitan areas were examined, the researchers found that more than 40% of the necessary care was either lacking or simply incorrect. A variety of evaluation methods were used, and the strength of this important study lies not only in the number of subjects and wide geographic representation, but also in the breadth of medical conditions or clinical encounters reviews: well-child care (e.g., immunizations and physical examinations), acute medical problems (e.g., fever, upper respiratory tract infections, diarrhea), and chronic conditions (acne, asthma, and depression) were all studied.

Among the findings:

- Only 50% of children who were two years of age or older had received all recommended vaccinations. Since vaccinations are extraordinarily cost-effective, and since many of the diseases they prevent can only be partially treated and leave an affected child with much long-term morbidity, this is a particularly striking result.

- For young children with fever of unclear origin—a common symptom in daily practice often due to urinary tract infections that in turn can lead to chronic kidney damage or death— fewer than one in five had a urine culture performed. (Medical literature studies, done in practice settings, recommend that all very young children with fever without an obvious source have a urine culture performed.)

- For routine adolescent care, less than half of girls had laboratory testing for vaginal infection caused by an organism (*Chlamydia trachomatis*) that can lead to infertility or life-threatening complications during a later pregnancy.

- Among asthmatic children and adolescents, only about 45% received appropriate care.

Besides the unnecessary suffering in both the short and long run, the tragedy is that almost all of these necessary interventions cost but a few dollars.

To be sure, there are limitations to this first-of-its-kind study in the pediatric population: it was retrospective, depended on chart review (meaning that failure to find evidence of appropriate care might have been due to mere note-taking mistakes), and the children studied tended to be less healthy than most children (as evidenced by the fact that they were seen by doctors on a rather frequent basis; many children almost never see the doctor).

But while some of these potential pitfalls may apply, it is likely that the failure to deliver appropriate care was common and widespread. There is little reason to believe that the same sloppiness that is so well revealed in the Dartmouth study *doesn't* apply to children, and now we have the first robust evidence of that unpleasant reality. The study didn't even attempt to address the amount of *unnecessary* care delivered, but that too is likely to be found in the younger-than-Medicare-age population. As unpleasant as it is to conclude, the vast American health care system is, at great cost to individuals as taxpayers and as patients, failing to deliver the simple, effective treatments that extend life and, equally important, to extend life free of disease or suffering from the complications of common diseases. There is an almost inexplicable difference in the likelihood that one will receive appropriate, proven, inexpensive, and simple treatment for many common diseases. In short, we have reviewed some of the representative examples of the "underutilization" of cost-effective medical services. In the next chapter, we'll look at the problems created by overutilization.

NOTES

1. "Preference-Sensitive Care." A Dartmouth Atlas Project Topic Brief. (Hanover, NH: Center for the Evaluative Clinical Science, November 15, 2004), available at: http://www.darmouthatlast.org.
2. The careful reader will note that the vertical scale is a "log" scale meaning that each increment is factor of 10 bigger. So "2" on a log scale is 10 times larger than "1", and "3" is ten times larger still.
3. We really should emphasize the term 'appear' here. New mechanisms of beta-blockers are identified every year. One of the most recent mechanisms identified showed that the medication actually was able to improve the function of individual muscle heart cells!
4. Prophylactic medicine, being something that prevents disease or its recurrence.
5. Rita Mangione-Smith, Alison H. DeCristofaro, Claude M. Setodji, Joan Keesey, David J. Klein, John L. Adams, Mark A. Schuster, and Elizabeth A. McGlynn, "The Quality of Ambulatory Care Delivered to Children in the United States." *New England Journal of Medicine*, 357;15: 1515–1523.

CHAPTER 3

Nothing Exceeds Like Excess

FROM THE IN-DEPTH WORK of the Dartmouth group it is difficult to avoid the conclusion that there is a huge variation in the intensity of (and in the number of dollars spent in) medical care among the over-65-year-old population. Medical care expenditures in the United States probably topped $2 *trillion* for the first time in 2007, about 13% to 15% of the entire U.S. economy, depending on varying estimates in gross domestic product. If much of that money fails to improve the quality or quantity of life, then change is desperately needed. Indeed, it has been appreciated for some time that, despite spending more than twice as much per capita in the United States than in European countries and in Japan, overall life expectancy, infant mortality, and complications from common medical conditions are far worse in the United States.

Despite the macroeconomic evidence for a failing health care system, the bountiful funding of health care hasn't received much scrutiny. As a percentage of GDP, health care has grown every year since the 1950s save for a brief period in the late 1980s, when the introduction of managed care plans and health maintenance organizations briefly put the brakes on the rate of rise of medical payments, which traditionally exceeded inflation by a factor of 2 or 3. Insurance companies were able to temporarily negotiate contracts with physicians and hospitals that, in turn, led to squeezing out some of the excess capacity in expensive hospital beds. In addition, a few striking studies—for example, one showing that the use of athroscopic procedures for evaluating and treating chronic degenerative knee pain were no better than doing nothing at all—perhaps stayed the hands of orthopedic surgeons anxious to perform another lucrative surgical intervention. But the paring back in the rate of growth of health care expenditures was temporary. Today we are back to the same yearly rise in medical costs that was experienced throughout most of the 1970s, 1980s, and 1990s. Yet, despite the spiraling costs, as anyone who reads a newspaper from time to time knows, at any given moment about 40 to 50 million Americans lack health insurance. Almost all of these uninsured individuals are under the age of 65 because Medicare provides for most of the health care needs of the elderly.

Without simple prevention and primary care treatment of common conditions, serious complications like heart attacks and stroke inevitably erupt, and they force the suddenly critically ill individual to the emergency room (ER). ERs serve as the refuge of last resort for very ill people without insurance, but they are very expensive places to get health care that might have otherwise been unnecessary. And, because ERs are staffed by physicians who are generally not familiar with the patients they are suddenly forced to take care of, costs mount quickly during an episode of care as tests are repeated for lack of access to a paper chart that might be in another ER—or perhaps a long forgotten physician's office—miles or a whole continent away.

So emergency rooms are the source of a common problem in medicine: unnecessary or expensive testing and treatments (or both), in part because of a lack of information on a given patient's history.

As we explored in the last chapter, given that physicians in one part of a city or one part of the country are five to ten times as likely to employ some expensive medical procedure—at least among the elderly—with no demonstrable benefit, one conclusion is unavoidable: they can't all be right. Failure to get the right information is clearly a reason for this variation, but, as we will show in this chapter, failure to *use* information correctly is a much bigger root cause.

Let's look at the typical coronary patient who is admitted to the hospital with chest pain and who is found to have a "blockage" of one or more coronary arteries. We already know that the probability of use of coronary artery angioplasty and also coronary artery bypass is extremely variable across the country. We also know that the chances of a patient receiving aspirin to prevent a second heart attack (including one that might occur shortly after a first heart attack) vary enormously. But what if we ask this question: is there a correlation between overall intensity of care as measured by invasive, expensive procedures and the probability of also getting the simple stuff, like baby aspirin? The answer is, once again, striking because it is unexpected: in the very areas of the country where a coronary patient is most likely to receive lots of high-tech interventions such as angioplasty they are *least* likely to get aspirin.

The data from the Dartmouth study among Medicare patients is shown in Figure 3-1. Of patients who receive the *least* intensive service ("quintile" number 1, the lowest cost of the five groups), about 85% receive aspirin (which costs only a penny or two a day). As the intensity of service increases (quintiles 2 through 5), the likelihood that the cardiologist or internist will prescribe aspirin drops (the green boxes indicate the average number, represented by the horizontal line, and the uncertainty or statistical deviation from the mean is represented by the triangular box). The absence of overlap of the boxes from one quintile to the next tells the statistician that the differences are indeed significant and not just a statistical fluke.

So, in quintile 5—the most expensively treated group of coronary patients whose care is fully twice as pricey as those in quintile 1—the chance of getting aspirin is reduced from 85% to 70%. There is not a

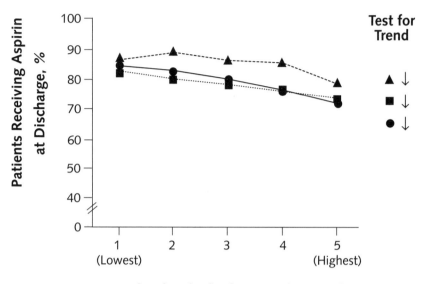

FIGURE 3-1. Percentage of coronary patients receiving aspirin prescriptions at discharge, grouped by total intensity or expenditure of other services. Intensity is ranked from lowest (1) to highest (5) and is based on cost and number of invasive procedures performed in patients who have had heart attacks.

cardiologist in the country who would deny that aspirin is the single most effective drug for preventing the recurrence of coronary atherosclerosis and much more effective than expensive cholesterol drugs.

It turns out that the same findings apply for beta blockers—which generally cost about 25¢ per day—are the next most effective drugs in preventing heart attacks. They, too, are *least* likely to be prescribed for the patients receiving the *greatest* amount of expensive interventional procedures. Based on effectiveness, just about everyone should receive beta blockers (save for those who cannot tolerate them), but only about 45% of heart attack patients leave the hospital with a prescription for these life-saving medications.

It's not just the specialists who make errors of underutilization and overutilization. In the primary care world, simple measures are often overlooked.

Consider the large number of people who are treated annually for pneumonia, many requiring hospitalization. It is a good bet that if you are diagnosed with a serious case of pneumonia—one so bad that a large portion of your lungs is incapable of absorbing oxygen from the air because of fluid and pus filling the tiny air sacs that have become infected—you'll receive excellent care in the emergency room and intensive care unit. You might even require a respirator, the services of a pulmonary specialist and intensive care unit nurses around the clock, special antibiotics, and then a long period of rehabilitation, should you be fortunate enough to survive.

Indeed, pneumonia in the elderly or near-elderly is a leading cause of death, and the two most common forms of pneumonia—from the virus called influenza and from a bacteria known as pneumococcus— can be almost completely prevented by vaccination. The vaccines are cheap, proven, and ubiquitously available. Indeed, for the Medicare population, the federal government makes the vaccines available for free (for just about no cost). But what if we look at the 306 HRRs in the United States and ask, "What percentage of enrollees are immunized against pneumococcus in any given two-year period?" The graph, as shown in Figure 3-2 is eerily similar to what we have seen before.

Several medical facts underscore the importance of the information in this graph. First, pneumococcus vaccine need be given only once (or at most twice) during a lifetime. Assuming that most people live to an age of 80 and don't, in general, even get an offer to receive the vaccine until about age 65, there is a 20-year window for receiving the vaccine. On average, as the graph shows, in any two-year period (or 10 "windows" of 2 years each), only 4% of the eligible population receives a vaccine against one of the most common mortal infectious diseases in the United States. In aggregate, taken over a 20-year pe-

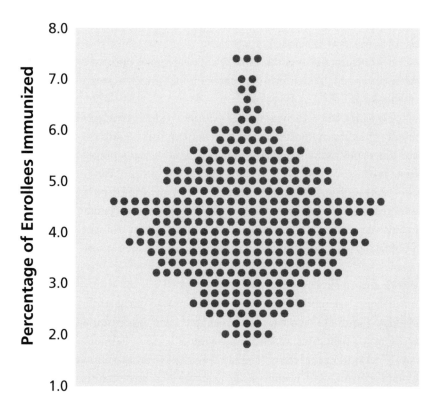

FIGURE 3-2. Percentage of Medicare enrollees who received immunization against pneumococcal pneumonia at least once in a two-year period (1995–1996).

riod, only about half of the population of elderly receives their once-in-a-lifetime pneumococcus vaccine.

The graph also shows that, in some parts of the county, coverage is about seven times better than in other parts of the country. In other words, your chance of getting this life-saving vaccine when it matters is between about 15% and 90%. There is simply no excuse for that because the vaccine has no serious side effects (for example, it cannot cause pneumococcus) and reactions to the vaccine are almost unheard of.

With influenza vaccine, the results are even worse—partly because, unlike the pneumococcus vaccine, influenza vaccine has to be given yearly (or at least every other year) to be effective because the influenza virus tends to mutate a bit from year to year, requiring a slight variation in the vaccine to afford protection. Put another way, while it is relatively easy—even for poor people who show up at ERs with advanced, life-threatening pneumonia—to get treatment in intensive care units at costs of well over $2,000 per day, the majority of elderly individuals never receive either a one-time pneumococcus vaccine nor their yearly flu vaccine. The cost of the latter two vaccinations is at most a few dollars per person, and in many places completely free.[1]

Thus, it is easy to see that in the United States too much of the expensive interventions are done and too little of the extremely beneficial, inexpensive prescriptions. The conclusion is the same, independent of medical specialty, although of course it is most noticeable (both in the pocketbook and in terms of quality of life) in the specialties that have the largest number of interventional tools and the largest number of patients with disease that falls into their specialties: cardiology and radiology lead the way by far because reimbursement levels for services in these specialties are very high.

We would note that, since the diseases on which we have data from the Dartmouth study affect people in their forties, fifties, and early sixties as well as the Medicare population, it is highly likely that precisely the same conclusions apply to all age groups afflicted by common diseases such as atherosclerosis, degenerative arthritis, and most types of cancer. We'll comment further on these specific disease entities in subsequent chapters. And now it is time to ask, "What might explain these scientifically indefensible practices?"

MORE ROOM AT THE INN MEANS MORE TREATMENT

Wennberg and his associates attempted to understand the dissimilarities in medical care across the United States for common conditions that *may* in some—but not all—circumstances require expending large amounts of medical resources. Because the researchers had only retrospective data, they had to formulate an explanatory hypothesis and then test it with mathematical models. The techniques they used are well accepted, falling into a branch of mathematics called "inferential" statistics, but they were acutely aware that merely showing a correlation does not prove causation. Thus, they had to formulate a reasonable hypothesis and then test their mathematical model in all areas of the country, looking to see if it applied widely and knowing that, if it in fact did, they most likely had a solid hypothesis that could shed light on the underlying root causes.

Here is what they found: the amount of money spent is directly related to the supply of physicians and the supply of hospital beds. This part of their study involves a bureaucratic-sounding term known as "the rate of care dependent on the supply." Let's break that term down into two pieces.

When the study refers to "supply," they mean, in this case, the limited amount of health care available in a given area. That's the supply of hospitals—in particular, hospitals that specialize in invasive, expensive, and very, very lucrative surgical procedures. It also counted the following:

- The number of doctors who performed the invasive procedures.

- The number of skilled registered nurses.

- The availability of pharmacies stocking and dispensing the specific medications related to the procedures.

- The number of available physical therapists.

Now, when the study talks about "rate," it means how often one of these gold-plated procedures are actually performed. So the study term measures the relationship of the available kind of care to the number of times that it's actually performed.

It is important to note that correlating on measurement with another does not *necessarily* imply—let alone prove—a specific causation. For example, if healthcare costs go up as the number of physicians per capita in a community increase, it may be because the population is, on average, more ill than in surrounding communities hence attracting physicians in the first place to care for them. One would be reassured, or at least unsurprised, that total costs would be higher. The Dartmouth researchers realized that it would be necessary to take into account—in a very rigorous and careful way—the severity of illness, age, gender, average education, socio-economic status, and other variables identified over the past 40 or 50 years to affect the outcomes of just about any medical problem one can name. Thus, the results presented in the Dartmouth reports reflect, to the best extent possible, an "average" patient, where the factors that can otherwise magnify the need for more intensive care of a simple medical problem (e.g., a respiratory infection that almost always resolves on its own or requires a short course of antibiotics) or one that is much more complex (e.g., multiple obstructions in the coronary arteries, which sometimes requires surgery to relieve the life-threatening reduction in blood flow to the heart and then long-term management of cholesterol levels and blood pressure to try to prevent recurrence).

The Dartmouth researchers began by evaluating treatment of acute diseases and decompensation of chronic diseases to see how likely it was across all of the HRRs in the United States that hospitalization would result *after* adjusting for the severity of illness and the other relevant factors on disease outcome listed above.

The Dartmouth researchers looked specifically at a group of diseases called "ambulatory care sensitive" conditions—that is, medical disorders for which there is general agreement that, if properly managed in the outpatient (nonhospital) setting, in most cases they should not advance to the point where hospitalization should be required (although on occasion they doubtless do). Some of these conditions are[2]:

- Serious skin infections (sometimes called "cellulitis").

- Asthma.

- Chronic lung disease such as emphysema or related condition.

- Chronic heart failure.

- Dehydration (particularly in the very old).

- Pneumonia.

- Urinary tract infection.

- Acute complications of diabetes.

Figure 3-3 would seem to indicate that the more hospital beds that are available, the more likely it is that a given individual would be admitted for a common condition that in general could be prevented in the first place, and the more likely it is that a hospitalization will take place.

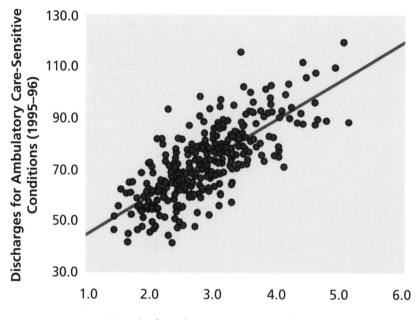

FIGURE 3-3. Is availability of health care related to use of health care?

Other explanations are possible, of course. For example, perhaps the very same places where lots of hospital beds were available happened to be in poor areas (or cities) of the country and, since poor people often don't get medical care until terrible complications of common problems compel them, maybe the increased hospitalization rate is really causally related to the level of poverty. But that explanation begins quickly to fall flat. Wealthier communities tend to be the places where there are more hospital beds per capita, and since the correlation in Figure 3-3 holds across the entire country, it would seem that the availability of this particular medical service—skilled nursing care in a hospital—per se drives hospital admissions.

A similar relationship between the number of physicians and the total cost also obtains, and the same counterarguments can be made. But once again, physicians (and subspecialty physicians in particular) tend to locate in wealthy parts, communities, or cities of the country, and hence it seems that the number of physicians per capita, rather than the actual severe disease burden per capita, drives the utilization of resources.

THE DOLLAR COST OF VARIABILITY IN THE LATTER YEARS OF LIFE

Dartmouth researchers have also found that the amount spent per patient varied from about $25,000 to well over six figures during the last two years of a patient's life; there were similar variations among patients not expected to die but with potentially "expensive" diseases, such as coronary artery obstructions. That's almost a five-fold variation, and keep in mind that, since the starting point is the $25,000 price tag, the high-end facilities were spending over $100,000 per patient.

And, once again, it probably wouldn't surprise you to find out that, in general, the higher-expense areas tend to be wealthier areas, and the lower-expense areas tend to be poor. That is, the more wealthy the community is, the more money was spent to keep the patient alive in the last two years of their life; more procedures were done, more drugs ordered and swallowed or injected, and more nurse care or physical therapy ordered.

However, there is another surprise buried in the study's numbers. In the cases where the most money and the most care were lavished on the luckier (or at least wealthier) patients, the outcomes were slightly *worse* than in the poorer areas: specifically, the survival rate of the patients was actually slightly lower in the areas where the most money was spent.

You might think this is counterintuitive. But there is actually a reasonable explanation for the result. The Dartmouth study has proven, within reasonable statistical confidence, that the higher expenditure areas simply have more doctors assigned to the average patient's case and that, when there are more doctors per capita, other unintended consequences arise.

MANY CAPTAINS, ONE SHIP

If there are more doctors, the patient's care tends to get fractionated. Many people are making decisions, communicating via hard-to-read notes in the patient's chart (and occasionally by phone call, but multiple phone calls simply take too much time). Nobody is really in charge, even though ostensibly there is supposed to a physician of record, or an attending or primary care physician, who has the responsibility of coordinating care. Coordinating care is much more easily said than implemented. What if two or three subspecialists disagree? Can one expect a typical family doctor to resolve the impasse? Frequently—though the numbers are hard to come by—the large team of well-intentioned caregivers muddles through, with medications started by one doctor, changed by a second, and then perhaps stopped or changed again by a third.

Thus, one reason that outcomes don't improve with more medical services is that a given individual will see many more physicians with ever more narrow specialty talents in the high-expense areas and see them more often than they will in the low-expense areas. There isn't a captain of the team. There are instead many captains, each of whom is pursuing a narrow area of interest but not communicating well with the others.

It is common knowledge among doctors that it is tough to have regular communication with two or three others caring for the same patient, who also have heavy patient caseloads and hectic schedules. Imagine what happens when five or six or seven physicians try to communicate with each other!

As you add doctors, the number of interactions between them immediately skyrockets. In mathematics, this type of phenomenon is commonly referred to as the "n-factorial problem," and it describes in precise numerical terms the number of interactions that might take place when one doctor tries to fully coordinate his or her thoughts, recommendations, or actions with the other doctors on a team taking care of just one patient. "N,factorial" means to take a number—in this case the number of doctors involved in given patient's care—and then multiply it by the next smaller number, then the next smaller number, then the next smaller number until you get to 1.

So, for example, if there are three doctors on a case, you can figure out how many interactions have to take place to keep all of them informed by thinking of them as three factorial: $3 \times 2 \times 1 = six$. In other words, six interactions have to take place for all three doctors to know what the other doctors are doing.

Now, see how quickly this gets out of control with even more doctors trying to stay "in the loop" when it comes to a patient's care. If there are four doctors, then it's $4 \times 3 \times 2 \times 1$, which is suddenly 24—quadruple the communications burden of having only three doctors. And if there are five doctors? It's a jaw-dropping 120 interactions—and that's if the five doctors are even aware of each other and actively trying to keep each other informed on the patient's care.

So you can see that, the more doctors that are involved, the number of interactions among those doctors that *ought* to be taking place grows far faster than exponentially. And in the fast-paced, time-limited world of modern mass medicine, these interactions simply do not take place. There just isn't enough time, and it is easy to see how adding just one more opinion can take a difficult management situation and render it impossible to control. This phenomenon may explain why outcomes are worse as the intensity of services—inevitably reflected in the number of doctors involved—increases.

FOLLOWING THE MONEY

By and large, almost all hospital beds are filled almost all the time because that's the way the hospital wants the situation. That's partially because hospitals have tried to cut down on the overhead costs because it's expensive to maintain a bed that's empty. A hospital bed, it should be noted, is a much different and more complex item than the bed you might have in your bedroom.

Hospitals have to have a nurse to staff it and you have to provide power. And you have to keep it and the rooms pristinely clean. So there's always pressure from the top to get rid of overage, but, once you have a bed, administrators want to have it filled because, when a bed is occupied, it is a lucrative source of income from insurance carriers and Medicare. Hospital care and its associated services from radiology, the laboratory, other available diagnostic services, such as ultrasound machines and consultants, can easily generate thousands of dollars a day of income for the hospital (assuming there is someone to pay the bill).

This phenomenon is probably best illustrated by the rise of the so-called *boutique* or *specialty* hospital. These special hospitals generally fall into three basic niches:

- Cardiac disease centers

- Orthopedic disease specialists (mostly elective knee replacements for osteoarthritis)

- Cancer centers

You'll never see a boutique hospital specializing in the treatment of elderly people with pneumonia. That's not because pneumonia isn't dangerous, even though, as a matter of fact, it is one of the biggest killers of the elderly. You won't see a pneumonia center because that's simply not very lucrative. There are lot of costs involved in the treatment and little in the way of diagnostic testing that is needed.

Contrast that with your local orthopedic specialty hospital offering both inpatient and outpatient surgical procedures such as hip and knee replacements or arthroscopy of the knee for athletes who have sustained some injury. If you can operate on relatively healthy people who simply have bum knees, you can make a lot of money without much risk of complications. Better yet, you won't even have to spend a lot of money taking care of them because generally healthy people— that is, those with coexisting conditions (usually called "comorbidities" in the medical literature)—heal well and are out of the hospital quickly.

These specialty hospitals are, to an almost universal extent, owned by physicians. They go by the name of physician-owned specialty hospitals (POSHs). According to a report to Congress filed in 2005,[3] these hospitals:

- Do not have lower costs for Medicare patients than community hospitals, although their patients have shorter lengths of stay.

- Treat patients who are generally less severe cases and concentrate on particular diagnosis-related groups (DRGs), some of which are relatively more profitable.

- Tend to have lower shares of Medicaid patients than community hospitals.

Medicaid patients tend to be poorer than the average patient. So, what this report has shown is that POSHs "cherry-pick" the least ill, resulting in fewer complications with which the physicians must deal. At the same time, the POSHs fail to provide their fair share of charity or pro bono care. Since Medicare reimburses by diagnosis code and procedures performed, the patients admitted to POSHs who are less ill to start off with and for whom the physician can justify a highly reimbursed procedure or two—say, a cardiac catherization followed by a bypass operation—result in high profits to they physicians who invest in the facilities. It is little wonder that they are springing up at an ever increasing rate across the country.

Unsurprisingly, you won't find POSHs for the treatment of many primary care problems like pneumonia, diabetes, or emphysema. The reason is simple: it's not lucrative. In fact, hospital admissions for complications of common primary care problems is typically a money *loser* for most hospitals. Caring for patients on whom specialized procedures are *not* done means that hospitals stand at best only a so-so chance of breaking even. Multiply that over the number of people who'd be admitted to such a hospital and it would be only a matter of time before the center started operating at a major loss.

WHAT IS TO BE DONE?

It is clear that in the modern-day practice of medicine in America, the opportunity to use inexpensive, simple, safe, effective treatments and preventative measures is often missed. At the same time, extremely expensive, dangerous procedures of much less certain effectiveness are performed almost at the whim of physicians.

The wise analysts poring over the data in the Dartmouth study offer a solution to the documented excesses. They recommend that one way to control costs and variability in care is that physicians adopt what is called "preference sensitive care." What does this phrase mean? In areas where there are choices—because we don't know what the best single choice is—the patient's preference rather than the physician's preference should dictate the care in the areas of greatest uncertainty. Put another way, in those circumstances where the benefits to using a particular procedure are possible but far from guaranteed—indeed, they may make a bad situation much worse—the options and risks should be thoroughly discussed with the patient. Some time should be allowed to pass for the patient to think and ask questions, and then the decision should be made, jointly with the physician providing the best data *and* the clearest possible description of the uncertainties to the patient.

For example, in early-stage breast cancer, the traditional teaching up until perhaps 15 years ago was that there were only two legitimate treatments for breast cancer. These were a pair of unsavory choices:

- A full mastectomy, meaning removal of the entire breast.

- A radical mastectomy, meaning removal of the breast and the underlying muscle tissue.

We now know that other options, such as just removing the cancerous lump, or radiating the lump—a so-called lumpectomy or breast-sparing surgery—is just about as effective as a radical mastectomy. And it results in far less disfigurement and far less "morbidity"—that is, suffering. One example of the reduction in morbidity would be the lessening in the swelling of the arms because a simple lumpectomy with removal of a few lymph nodes (to determine with reasonable certainty whether the cancer has spread beyond the breast or not) does not compromise drainage of fluid from the arm that almost inevitably results from radical mastectomy and complete lymph node dissection. Given the choice, almost all women with early-stage breast cancer choose lumpectomy, reducing both complications and cost.

While we'll discuss prostate cancer in more detail in a subsequent chapter, in the case of males who may have the disease, there are essentially four options for its treatment. For the moment, we'll define prostate cancer now as the presence of abnormal cells on a biopsy, but, as will be seen later, there remains a vast disagreement over whether abnormal cells in the prostate gland do, in fact, constitute a disease (let alone cancer) that can lead to death or even compromise an otherwise healthy life. That's because these abnormal cells may or may *not* ever cause any problems outside the prostate, such as spreading malignantly to the bones or to other organs in the body.

Surprising as it may be to most readers, physicians cannot predict with high confidence which patients with abnormal-looking cells in the prostate will develop *metastatic* prostate cancer, which is the complication from prostate cancer otherwise remaining within the prostate gland itself that kills patients. It's not the little lump in the prostate gland, just like it's not the little lump in the breast, that kills you. It's the metastasis—spreading to other parts of the body—that kills you. Because of these uncertainties, it's reasonable to offer choices to individuals. One of these choices should always be doing nothing. (Note that this is unacceptable in breast cancer because we know that, in the vast majority of cases, it's nearly certain to be a progressive disease that eventually metastasizes.)

But prostate cancer may not be progressive; indeed, we know that the vast majority of males harboring prostate cancer will either never know it or, if they do, not suffer from metastatic disease. One procedure is to radiate the prostate gland over the course of a few days. This is done with an external X-ray beam, which is relatively simple to do because you can radiate the prostate gland coming in at multiple angles. This ends up concentrating the radiation in the prostate gland, so that the side effects are usually small, though the cost is a little high.

Second, one can implant seeds of radioactive material directly into the prostate gland that spread radiation out over an area of about one centimeter in length. So the prostate gland literally gets cooked with radiation, but usually no other tissue gets damaged.

Another option is to remove the prostate gland in its entirety—a procedure called "radical prostatectomy." Unfortunately, while one can be reasonably assured that radical prostatectomy does, indeed, remove all prostate cancer in the prostate gland we can't detect the spread of a small number of cells of prostate cancer, say 10 or 100 of them. Therefore, even a radical prostatectomy sometimes fails to cure the cancer. Two, three, or five years later, the patient can wind up with a sudden fracture of the femur because there have been prostate cancer cells growing in that bone since the time they had their prostate removed.

And radical prostatectomy comes at a price: the patient may be impotent following the procedure or suffer from urinary incontinence, at least in part because the nerves that control erection in the male and also lower bladder function may be damaged by the procedure.

From what little we know about prostate cancer—and "little" is a correct characterization—other than doing nothing, radical prostatectomy is *probably* the most effective of the three proactive options, but it comes with the highest likelihood of postoperative side effects. And, as already noted, it's not clear who among the many hundreds of thousands of men found each year to harbor prostate cancer cells will actually benefit from any of these procedures, for indeed most men who have prostate cancer "diagnosed" based on a biopsy of the gland do not have a disease that will actually harm them. They will die "with" prostate cancer cells in their prostate and not "because" of prostate cancer.

. . . AND THE PATIENT'S PREFERENCES

In the face of uncertainty, what researchers have found at least preliminarily, is that an informed patient choice—in the case of breast cancer for women and prostate cancer for men—results in better outcomes. Patient preference results not only in a better outcome usually measured as quality of life, but also in a dramatic decrease in the costs. In the case of prostate cancer, if you do a radical prostatectomy on everybody with prostate cancer, not only is that a very expensive procedure, which rewards the urologist very well, there are complications that require chronic care afterward.

So the cost arises not just from the initial large sum paid to the urologist in the hospital for the radical prostatectomy procedure. There is also long-term, chronic suffering in about 30% of patients who receive a radical prostatectomy. (It's much less in patients who receive external beam therapy or seed implantation, but the benefits may be less as well; research is still being conducted on this question.)

And, of course, the risks of short-term side effects are virtually zero in terms of people who undergo so-called "watchful waiting." This phrase simply means that the decision is to not do anything about this prostate cancer unless the number of cells in the prostate increase abnormally or appear to be growing more aggressively as seen under the microscope. When the possible complications stemming from more aggressive treatment include, but are not limited to, incontinence and impotence, the option to watch and wait should be included in the patient's suite of options.

. . . AND THE DOCTOR'S PREFERENCES

Almost anyone who has dealt with physicians has noticed that there remains a certain paternalism in medicine. Another way this manifests itself is in how commonly the preference of the physician gets imposed on the patient. That preference appears to be especially true when surgery is involved, and it is something against which every well educated patient should guard. This will be ever more true as yet additional options become available for the treatment of prostate cancer—which is far more likely to be a pathological curiosity than a disease.

If past is prologue, the new procedures will likely be abused rather than used properly.

If past is prologue, it appears new procedures or treatments will be rapidly implemented by the medical community before the actual benefits and risks are well defined. Since performing these procedures often results in a large payment to the physician—usually a surgeon as opposed to a primary care doctor—one unavoidable, uncomfortable hypothesis to explain the premature, wide-spread use of new technologies is that the financial incentive is so great, the physician may lose his objectivity in deciding or recommending a particular treatment when there are several other, perhaps less expensive or remunerative options, available.

Physicians, like any humans, may rationalize their recommendations by asserting that they are doing what they believe to be in the patient's best interest. But given the all-but-incontrovertible data we have already seen on how good outcomes are often inversely related to intensity of service and cost, and the extreme variations in use of a plethora of invasive, expensive procedures for the same disease types across the country, it is hard to ignore the possibility that the lure of higher financial reward drives some of physicians' decision-making.

This is an emotionally charged topic, and no professional—physicians included—tolerate the implication of taking advantage of a patient's illness for personal finance gain. Summarizing their many decades of research into the difficult-to-justify variations in medical care, the Dartmouth researchers address the issue this way:

> There is unwarranted variation in the practice of medicine and the use of medical resources in the United States. There is underuse of effective care, misuse of preference-sensitive care, and overuse of supply-sensitive care.
>
> - Underuse of most kinds of effective care (such as the use of beta-blockers for people who have had heart attacks and screening of diabetics for early signs of retinal disease) is very common even in hospitals considered among the "best" in the country—including some academic medical centers. The causes of underuse include discontinuity of care (which tends to grow worse when more physicians are involved in the patient's care) and the lack of systems that would facilitate the appropriate use of these services.
>
> - Misuse of preference-sensitive care refers to situations in which there are significant tradeoffs among the available options. Treatment choices should be based on the patient's own values (such as the choice between mastectomy and lumpectomy for early-stage breast cancer); but often they are not. Misuse results

from the failure to accurately communicate the risks and benefits of the alternative treatments, and the failure to base the choice of treatment on the patient's values and preferences. [Emphasis added.]

- Overuse of supply-sensitive care is particularly apparent in the management of chronic illness (such as admitting patients with chronic conditions such as diabetes to the hospital, rather than treating them as outpatients). The cause is an overdependence on the acute care sector and a lack of the infrastructure necessary to support the management of chronically ill patients in other settings.

. . . [Our] most important finding . . . was the striking contrast between need for surgery as defined by physicians and need as defined by *patient preferences* [emphasis added].

. . . There is evidence that the amount of care that would be demanded under shared decision making might be substantially less than is currently being provided. . . . What it is safe to conclude . . . is that current patterns of practice do not reflect demand based on patient preferences, and that geographic variations in rates of surgery that reflect physician practice style will persist until patients are actively involved in the decision process and there are incentives for physicians to adopt shared decision making."[1]

And therein we believe lies a big piece of the solution to spiraling health care costs. When the benefits of a given treatment or procedure remain unproven (although theoretically desirable), the doctor should think first, talk second, talk with the patient again, and then talk one more time before doing something. In the case of prostate cancer, when patients get past the shock of hearing the word "cancer" and learn that in their particular circumstance it is unlikely that the finding of abnormal cells in their prostate will do them any harm, they often decide to do nothing. Partially, the decision depends on a given patient's risk-taking preference: do I want to live with the uncertainty of dying because of prostate cancer or with the possibility that the therapy will cause chronic side effects that will make my remaining life unpleasant? Partially, it depends on whether or not something else—like preexisting heart disease or diabetes—is more likely to be the cause of death than prostate cancer.

The Dartmouth study is a landmark effort in health care research, touching on almost all important aspects of services that most of us take for granted as being science based. From the work of Wennberg and his associates, we've learned that—at least for the Medicare population—many hundreds of billions of dollars are spent every year without good justification and that, despite ever increasing budgets, the amounts only get larger.

Even more important, it is probably the case not only that these large but still limited resources are probably doing nothing to improve the quality of life and may well be damaging it, but also that the preferences of patients are, to a large extent, ignored. While it is clear that people with serious diseases are frightened and look to their physicians to do the right things, there can be no other conclusion than that in many circumstances the right things are simply not done. It is very likely that the findings in the Medicare population reflect wildly varying decision making in health care for younger people as well.

It is little wonder that every health care planner—from academics and government officials to CEOs of large HMOs—have the Dartmouth reports on their desks. But most physicians have never even heard about it. Ask your doctor about it sometime to find out for yourself.

NOTES

1. It will probably come as no surprise to readers that only about 35% of physicians and nurses receive a yearly influenza vaccine. And since they are taking care of patients, they can literally *transmit* influenza from one patient to another if they become ill—something that the vaccine almost completely prevents.
2. For readers interested in more detail, see Nancy T. McCall, Sc.D., Erica Brody, M.P.H., et al. "Investigation of Increasing Rates of Hospitlization for Ambulatory Care Sensitive Conditions Among Medicare Fee for Service Beneficiaries: Final Report." RTI International. CMS Contract No. 500–00–0029, Task Order No. 9. June 2004. Available at: http://www.cms.hhs.gov/Reports/Downloads/McCall_2004_3.pdf.
3. Report to the Congress: "Physician-owned specialty hospitals." (Washington, DC: Medicare Payment Advisory Commission, March 2005).

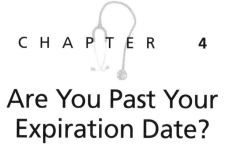

C H A P T E R   **4**

Are You Past Your
Expiration Date?

LIFE SPAN IN GENERAL has probably increased as a result of better nutrition and a far lower propensity for accidents. This happened when humans transitioned from the hunter-gatherer mode, which was the rule until about 10,000 years ago, and over to an agriculturally based existence. Food became more abundant, more reliable, and probably less associated with disease pathogens.

Make no mistake about it: the vast majority of increase in life expectancy beyond the mid-thirties has nothing to do with the latest technologies in modern medicine. But it has everything to do with better nutrition, avoiding accidents, and preventing exposure to infectious disease, either via vaccination or simply by living in protected environments, like houses and offices. A longer life span has even come from our ability to coordinate mass sanitation in a cultural sense, from regularly throwing out the trash to washing our hands before preparing food.

THE PRICE OF LIVING PAST YOUR EXPIRATION DATE

But living longer comes with a price because the cells in our body and in virtually every organ system have a limited number of reproduction cycles. In this chapter, we show that, while modern medicine has doubtless relieved much mortality from trauma and acute illness, chronic illness—which by definition never occurred when life spans were limited by environmental factors—generally defies much of the effort to combat it.

It turns out that on any given day, somewhere between a third and a half of people over the age of 45 walking down the street have some nagging complaint—a sore shoulder, a painful back, a bout of insomnia, perhaps a chronic cough—that leaves them feeling far from well. Sometimes, of course, there is a clear explanation for these problems such as moving furniture around the house the previous day. And, for smaller segments of that rather large portion of the middle-aged and older population that isn't feeling entirely well, there may be something very serious going on: an undiagnosed cancer that has metastasized to a bone to explain the back pain or pneumonia (the source is often unknown) to explain the cough. But for the majority of people feeling out of sorts on any given day, the cause is either never identified and the unpleasant sensations merely melt away. And if they don't, most people seek medical attention.

In this chapter, we adopt the medical terminology "symptom" when referring to the complaints or discomforts that individuals feel. Primary care doctors see the vast majority of patients whose symptoms bring them to the clinic or hospital. Even though much of the time discomfort in the joints or muscles or aching in the abdomen disappear without an underlying cause ever being found, a significant portion of the time these symptoms can last for months or even years. Although the data is very hard to come by—since most medical studies are based on a firm or specific diagnosis—health care providers have gradually come to realize that long-standing complaints, which tend to be either musculo-skeletal or gastrointestinal in origin, are very common, and also very frustrating for both the patient and the physicians who treat them. Many readers will have experienced, or know someone who has experienced, a long period of discomfort accompanied by numerous diagnostic tests in an attempt to identify the root cause of chronic symptoms only to be told that the myriad of X-rays and blood tests are "normal."

Patients are sometimes told that they suffer from "fibromylagia" or irritable bowel syndrome, but these are just names for what the patient already knows too well: chronic neck and shoulder pain in the first case, abdominal bloating and perhaps intermittent diarrhea or constipation in the second. The underlying reason or "cause" remains unclear, and very often patients feel as if their healthcare provider doesn't take them seriously if no serious abnormality is found on an X-ray, scan, or blood test.

Within the medical community itself, arguments have raged for more than a decade over whether or not fibromyalgia is a true medical condition or instead is a manifestation of depression or poorly defined psychiatric disturbance. The phrase "medically unexplained or functional somatic symptoms" headlines hundreds of articles in the recent medical literature, and we don't pretend to be able to identify the causes of the symptoms described above which, while apparently not life-threatening, are consequential in terms of medical costs, time lost from work, and, most significant, the loss of enjoyment of many of the pleasures of life. But we do suggest that the aging process itself might hold the key: Clearly some people age much more gracefully and with fewer chronic symptoms than others, and we seek to broaden the discussion and our understanding of chronic unexplained symptoms by briefly summarizing the basic biology in our genes and an introduction to "degenerative" diseases, which will be examined in somewhat more detail later in this book.

THE BODY'S EXPIRATION DATE

It might come as a shock to those healthy 50- and 60-year-olds that the human body is designed to last only around 45 years. Some people say as little as 35, but, if you look at premodern man before or up to the agricultural revolution of about 10,000 years ago, the average life expectancy in males was about 45 and in women a little bit longer than that. And even with the advent of modern medicine, regularly achieving the age of 70 years was uncommon until the 1950s, which is part of the reason our social security system has the funding issues that it does. The increased longevity is hard to tie to the interventions of physicians; rather it seems to be related more to behavior changes, to the gradual egress from rural settings (where at the very least accidents of all kinds are much more likely on a per-person basis than in most urban settings), and to some serendipitous discoveries and practices.

Dental studies bear this out as well, as but one example. Some simple preventive measures, flossing and brushing, have been instrumental in keeping people over 40 from losing all of their teeth. Even despite flossing, brushing, and regular visits to the dentist, plenty of people lose teeth, and that too is a representation of the design life of the human body.

This brings us to the exact nature of disease. The word "disease" derives from the negation of satisfaction of one's health: dis-ease, or quite literally, *the lack of ease*. Some symptoms may have a cause external to the body; some symptoms may be a result of an abnormal response of the body to environmental stimulus; and some may have no known explanation other than the perception of the individual to the stresses of daily life. Reaction to stress is something that hasn't necessarily gotten better as civilization has moved from the subsistence existence of hunting, on to farming, and into the specialized division of labor that has freed most of us from having to worry about where our next sustenance will materialize from.

In the absence of clear explanations, symptoms can take on a political or advocacy dimension. And that has led various organizations to *find* a "disease" to allegedly explain symptoms with either somewhat more or somewhat less precision, but always with a political spin. For example—and an example that some may regard as extreme—the well-respected World Health Organization (WHO) has used a very strange, sliding-scale definition of disease in its definition of health. To the WHO, health is not merely the absence of disease, but also a "state of mind" or a level of satisfaction. How much satisfaction? Well, one must not be merely avoiding illness but in fact thriving—economically and socially and in political freedom.

Such abstract definitions have very fuzzy limits; indeed satisfaction, or freedom from discomfort, may be impossible to achieve. Rather than discuss the political and philosophical dimensions of such a debate, let's consider the symptoms that seems to affect almost all of us to one degree or another as we age.

First, let's consider what we call "degenerative" disease. Our ancestors of 10,000 to 15,000 years ago did not often experience this. They simply didn't live long enough to develop modern degenerative diseases. There are some very notable exceptions; for example, the mummified remains of Egyptian royalty who lived into their fifties or sixties show the presence of arthritis. We know this in almost all cases due to telltale changes in the bones. Obviously, we can't say nearly as much about the soft tissues because they aren't as well preserved. But the point is clear: in certain very pampered segments of even ancient societies a few people lived past the "design life" of somewhere in their mid-forties, and they suffered many of the same disorders that plague or even dominate many of our concerns over wellness in modern-day life.

Degenerative disease might be loosely defined as disorders in function that probably represent survival beyond the genetic design life of the human body. Now, this immediately leads us to questions of how well cells reproduce; when a cell—for example, a blood cell, a liver cell, or a kidney cell—begins to die, how well does it reproduce to replace itself. Some cells are even programmed to die after a certain period of time, a process known as cell *apoptosis*, possibly the basis of aging and equally possibly the evolved behavior of cells to prevent cancer—the uncontrolled growth and spread of cells.

Here's a bit more on how the body's design to prevent cancer may relate to aging and degenerative disease processes. We know that there are very clear genetic changes in the error-checking mechanism and in the actual structure of the genetic code. These changes suggests that DNA, even when it's well protected by the cellular membrane and the nuclear membrane, simply starts to wear out. By wearing out, we don't mean that it goes a little threadbare like the hall carpet. We mean that it develops mutations, and the error-checking mechanism for reproducing that DNA goes awry. This is most commonly associated with the deadliest forms of cancer, but it applies to many, many other conditions as well, including, in all probability, autoimmune disease.

So, degenerative disease can be conceived conceptually as any disease that our predecessors who died in their forties never experienced. It was extremely unusual to see degenerative arthritis, the wearing out of the cartilage of the joints, in the mummified remains of people who lived 10,000 to 15,000 years ago simply because they didn't live that long.

Unfortunately, we still don't know what sets the biological clock, what determines its speed, or what triggers many of its key events. In fact, one of the greatest advances in the science of aging is simply that we've managed to winnow the large potential number of causes to a relative handful, but we don't have any clear answers as to why the cells of the body stop repairing themselves and slowly start to die. Much controversy remains. The notions most widely accepted in mainstream science include:

1. *Free Radical Damage, also known as the Wear-and-Tear Theory:* This is the idea that changes associated with aging are the result of damage that accumulates over time, specifically the damage caused at a cellular level by particles known as free radicals. This is probably the most widely accepted belief among the lay public, insofar as it's kicked off a booming market in antioxidant nutrients, which claim to trap or otherwise eliminate free radicals and the damage they can cause. There is, unfortunately, little evidence that they perform as promised.

2. *Somatic Mutation Theory:* This is the biological theory that aging results from damage to the genetic integrity of the body's cells as a result of accumulated mutations, as DNA is copied and reproduced during cell division.

3. *Accumulative Waste Theory:* This is another biological theory of aging that points to a buildup of cells of waste products that presumably interferes with metabolism.

4. *Autoimmune Theory:* This is the idea that aging results from gradual decline in the immune system's ability to distinguish "foreign" matter (like infectious organisms) from "self" tissue. How the body makes the distinction in the first place is still a mystery; how it might *lose* that ability is even more obscure. However, the basic notion is that the immune system may, to some extent, lose this ability, leading to even earlier cell death or apoptosis.

5. *Error Accumulation, or Cellular, Theory:* This theory takes the view that aging can be explained largely by the changes in structure and function taking place in the cells of an organism, and is related to the Somatic Mutation Theory. It's also one of the most popular among cellular biologists because the current hypothesis is that clock speed and duration have to do with a genetic structure called the *telomere*. A telomere, as shown in Figure 4-1, is a region of highly repetitive DNA at the end of a linear chromosome that functions as a disposable buffer.

Ironically, telomeres first came into the eye of researchers via studies not of aging, but of cancer—one of the premier life shorteners. It was noted that, while telomeres in normal cells got slowly shorter and shorter over repeated divisions, the same was not true of cancerous cells. Cancerous tumors are able to reproduce infinitely, robbing the host body of nutrients and causing trauma and death to the body. It now appears that, at least in humans, tumors are able to achieve this cellular immortality by overexpressing *telomerase*. Telomerase is an enzyme that adds a specific DNA sequence to the end of DNA strands in the telomere regions.

Adding to the suspicion is that a sizable fraction of cancerous cells employ alternative lengthening of telomeres, involving the transfer of telomere tandem repeats—in essence, "swapping" telomeres. The mechanism by which this takes place is not fully understood because the exchange events are difficult to assess while the cells are undisturbed in the body. In either case, it appeared that if a cell's telomeres don't run out, neither will an organism's life span.

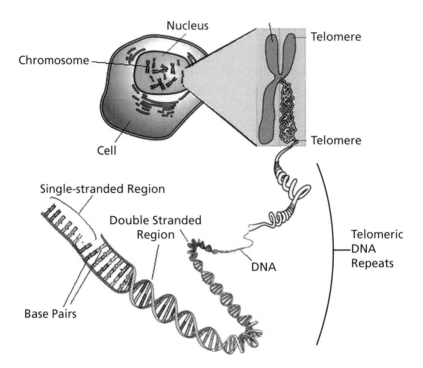

FIGURE 4-1. A drawing of a chromosome and a close-up of the telomere at the end.

DEADLY TURNOVER

Whether by shorter telomeres or other means, the reproductive capacity of cells to replace their own deaths eventually slows or comes to a halt. This is especially evident in cell types that "turn over" quickly: skin cells, gastrointestinal cells, and the cells that line any wet mucosal surface, such as in the mouth or in the stomach.

Therein probably lies the basis of degenerative diseases we start to experience in our fifties. For example, skin gets thin, dry, and crinkly, and it develops the many benign tumors (and sometimes malignant ones) that we see in older individuals all the time. Degenerative disease is really just a descriptive term that refers to the failure of cells in organs to accurately reproduce and therefore perpetuate their functionality.

Now, some humans appear to be far more susceptible to degenerative disease than others. We're all familiar with people who seem ageless, whereas others look much older than their actual age. Is this genetic in its basis or environmentally induced? The short answer is that we just don't know.

From the standpoint of individual organs, some seem relatively resistant to mutation-induced changes simply because their cells apparently last a long time without reproducing themselves. The brain is an example of an organ that really undergoes very little degenerative disease in the sense of the abnormal reproduction of cells. This because, once the brain reaches full maturity, its functional nerve cells, called *neurons*, don't reproduce at all; they just gradually die off without reproducing.[1]

One very benign effect of aging is when hair turns gray. Graying turns out to be due to the death of the melanin-producing cells in the root of the hair, which is really a specialized skin structure. The melanin-producing cells are actually thought to be fairly closely related to neurons!

On the other hand, rapidly reproducing cells—hair cells, skin cells, gastrointestinal cells—start to become susceptible to ever increasing numbers of genetic mistakes that are made in copying the DNA. This is probably the basis of the abnormal growth of cells, the unregulated growth of cells that we call cancer.

Abnormal genetic reproduction—sometimes called transcriptional errors (i.e., cumulative errors when newly minted genes become part of new cells)—almost inevitably lead to dysfunction in those cells. Some of these will naturally have a propensity, among other things, to not carry out their usual function but to grow in unconstrained fashion. And that is the start of a cancerous growth. As you might expect, the most common cancers by far occur in various organs or portions of organs where cells are reproducing rapidly: breast cancer, skin cancer, gastrointestinal cancer, and, in the case of smokers, lung cancer.

Where does this information leave the patient and the doctor who are struggling to deal with degenerative or age-related symptoms? Let's set aside natural variations that may provide insight into why some folks seem to age better than others. It is clear that the sociologic evolution of society has something to do with the challenges—moving from the depravations of living in a hunter-gatherer society to a more urban environment, which was originally plagued with poor sanitation in water and food supplies, and on again to modern most urban-based dwelling with clean water and a very safe and varied food supply. This progression has enabled most of us to expect to outlive the cells that make up the organs of our bodies and that have evolved to reproduce and replace themselves. Medicine has had little effect on the progress of much of degenerative disease that has supervened; we can't do much to slow (and certainly not reverse) common arthritis, dementia such as Alzheimer's disease, and cancer, to the extent that it is a manifestation of DNA mutations gone so far awry as to cause cells to proliferate wildly, damaging other cells often in distant organs—a topic we'll discuss in a subsequent chapter.

Joint replacements—not joint rejuvenation—is more or less all that we can offer to patients with worn-out knees and hips. This is certainly nothing to discount; many people who would otherwise be wheelchair bound or severely limited in function have been granted years of enjoyable life. And clearing blocked arteries has certainly prolonged the lifetimes of many. But these mechanical "fixes" are really a symptom of their own: a symptom of our failure to yet understand the fundamental nature of aging and the myriad of cellular processes that are altered with time. We can have some hope, now that the tools of molecular biology enable researchers to study DNA structure and function in exquisite detail, that we might be able to reverse or at least slow the aging process, but this remains a promise, not a realization.

As our society ages—and there is little doubt that the average age will increase worldwide as fewer children are born per female with increasing wealth—the costs and morbidity from degenerative disease will certainly increase. For the moment, remaining as active as possible on a regular basis and perhaps limiting stress while prudently avoiding becoming overweight—not easy to do in a world where food is usually ubiquitous and tempting—is about all one can do to slow the aging process. There are no medical miracles—like the discovery of antibiotics for infection—to point at, and one would do well to remain skeptical of claims of dietary supplements, megavitamins and the like to mitigate degenerative diseases. Finally, there is no evidence, in the absence of symptoms, that screening for degenerative diseases—MRI scans of joints, the heart, or the brain—provide actionable information that will alter the course of these now common scourges in modern society.

NOTES

1. Dartmouth Atlas Project Topic Brief, "Preference-Sensitive Care, November 2005. Available at www.dartmouthatlas.org.
2. On a related note, because neurons reproduce slowly, if at all, nerve damage to the brain or spinal cord is very difficult if not impossible to heal. For this reason, much stem cell research has been done to create new neurons in order to bridge neural gaps and cure Alzheimer's or help quadriplegics to walk again.

CHAPTER 5

Screening Out Common Sense

WHILE PROMOTIONS for prescription drugs predominate the airwaves, the advertisements touting the value of early screening seem to be a close second.

"Prevent disease before it occurs!"

"Detect cancer in its early curable stages, the smart choice of the man/woman today."

"Get yourself checked by a doctor—today!"

Sounds pretty good, doesn't it? After all, mom told us a long time a go that "an ounce of prevention is better than a pound of cure."

Except when it isn't true. Disease screening began to catch on in the 1980s in the primary care specialties of medicine: internal medicine, family practice, general practice. Like much of the rest of health care, delivery to the patient was put into widespread use well before the hypothesis was tested. There's no question that the concept is logical. After all, who can argue with preventing disease?

There's also no question that a *few* of the things that physicians do to try to keep their clientele out of trouble and out of the hospital do in fact work. But what's striking is how few of diagnostic tests make a difference and, when they do make a difference, how little difference they make.

HOW DOCTORS MAKE DECISIONS DURING CHECKUPS

Let's start with the most common of all traditional concepts: the annual physical exam. For as long as most people can remember, your family doctor encouraged you to have a yearly physical. This ritual, which is being paid for by insurance more and more rarely, involves first a detailed review of symptoms. These might include any of the following:

- Sensations you might be experiencing such as pain, fevers, or weight loss

- Behaviors that put you at risk for certain conditions—smoking, exercise regimen, dietary habits, and exercise

- Family history of various diseases, such as cancer or heart disease

- Medications you might be taking

This would be followed by poking and prodding to a greater or lesser extent, depending on the patience and beliefs of the doctor. Sometimes a skin growth might be discovered that turned out to be cancer. Occasionally, the doctor would elicit a history of blood in the stools, leading to further diagnostic tests that identified a polyp or even colon cancer at a curable stage. Or maybe the chest pain that occurs while climbing a few flights of stairs would lead to a diagnosis affecting the heart.

For a time, insurance companies encouraged their subscribers to go through this process. It seemed to make good business sense; after all, the annual physical might forestall much more expensive problems down the road, which meant more premiums for the company and fewer payouts. And who can fail to notice the front page story each year, when the president of the United States gets his annual physical exam at Bethesda Naval Medical Center? This story is usually complete with the obligatory picture of a dozen smiling doctors in their white uniforms, who invariably pronounce the nation's chief executive as "remarkably fit for a man of his age."

But we now know that it's pretty much all for naught. The president, while complaining about the ever rising cost of health care in the United States, is contributing to the spiraling expenditures via his own not-so-private exposé of intimate details of his examination. Make no mistake: there are a few things that doctors can do to fend off disease. But where most of us—physicians included—go wrong is when we fail to recognize one key fact. That annual physical and screening diagnostic tests are part of a process that, if handled incorrectly, can result in a worse outcome than doing nothing.

The screening process looks something like the flow chart in Figure 5-1. It looks simple, and in theory it is. But the connection between the step-by-step decisions and the key details of making them are rarely revealed in medical training or in textbooks. Consider the following details:

- The number of available "routine screening tests" has doubled every 5 years for the past 20 years. Most have proved to be worthless or, as we shall see, something closer to worse than worthless.

- The pressure on physicians to obtain screening tests has increased. The sources are advertisement from purveyors of the technology or, worse, physician-owners of diagnostic facilities, including, most recently, the owners of specialty ("boutique") hospitals.

- The outcomes from referral to specialist vary immensely, as already reviewed in the chapter on the Dartmouth study,

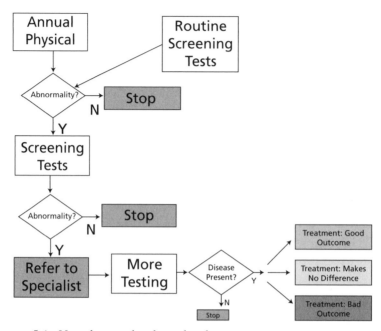

FIGURE 5-1. How doctors decide to do what.

which basically says, "Your chances of having an invasive diagnostic procedure or a therapeutic intervention that significantly improves your quality and quantity of life varies a great deal." And remember, on average, the outcomes are inversely related to how much service is provided; more is not better. There are exceptions, of course, and we'll tease them out in this chapter

- Finally, the lack of understanding by health care professionals themselves—physicians included—of the value of diagnostic tests leads to a resigned acceptance of patient demands (sometimes enforced by high-profile lawsuits). It's very hard to keep up if one hasn't the basic scientific knowledge to understand the screening tests, and most physicians simply don't understand them.

We'll begin by dealing with the last—and most fundamental—problem first in some detail.

WHAT "SENSITIVE" AND "SPECIFIC" MEAN

All diagnostic tests, without exception, have inherent error rates. No matter how good a test is, it isn't perfect. Even a test that is 99.99% accurate will on rare occasion give you a false negative—or a false positive. To know the implications of a test result for an individual patient, the physician must be knowledgeable about two pieces of information:

1. The sensitivity of the test.
2. The specificity of the test.

Let's look at each quality one at a time. *Sensitivity* is easy to understand. It's the chance (between 0 and 100%) that the test will be abnormal *if* the underlying disease is present. For example, if you or your child has a sore throat, the doctor may take a swab sample and perform a simple test called the "streptozyme assay," which works much like a home pregnancy test (although obviously for another purpose). An enzyme is secreted by the strep organism that can be readily detected by the streptozyme kit. Thus, if streptococcus (or, more accurately, the kind of strep called "Group A strep" that can cause serious disease) is present, the streptozyme test is almost always positive. We know from many studies that, if strep is present, the streptozyme test will be positive 95% of the time. We thus say, "The streptozyme test has a sensitivity of 95%." Another way of looking at this is that there is only a 5% chance that the test will be negative in the presence of streptococcus organisms in the throat.

Most doctors stop there and conclude, "That's a good test." But they would be wrong. What if the test is positive when the streptococcus organism is not present? That would mean that results of a positive test are less reliable and certainly harder to interpret.

This is where the concept of *specificity* arises. A test is said to be "highly specific" if it is positive *only* when the condition of concern is present. In the case of the streptozyme test, we know that about 15% of people have sore throats due to something other than streptococcus. Why? It usually turns out to be one of a myriad of viruses or occasionally one of several bacteria that are not very serious. Patients with these viruses or bacteria also have a positive streptozyme test when they go to their doctor complaining of a sore throat.

Physicians will say that the streptozyme test is "reasonably specific." Scientists who are a bit more quantitative say, "The streptozyme test has a specificity of 85%." Where did the "85%" come from? It comes from subtracting the 15% rate of falsely positive tests—that is, a positive test result when no strep is present—from 100%.

THE GOLD STANDARD IN STREP

Obviously we'd love to have perfect tests, which means 100% sensitive (never missing the presence of a given condition of concern) and 100% specific (meaning never overdiagnosing by saying a condition exists when it in fact does not). The tests that come closest are what physicians call the "gold standard." They include biopsies showing cancer of the lung, throat cultures showing the presence of streptococcus, and severe narrowing of an artery, as seen during an angiogram procedure. But tests of this level of accuracy are few and far between.

So what is a knowledgeable person to do with this information about sensitivity and specificity? We'll again consider the problem of the sore throat, where the physician's concern is the detection of the streptococcus organism. Detection is fairly important. If untreated, up to 3 out of 100 patients with strep can get a very serious complication, such as a throat abscess or rheumatic fever.

Let's say it's wintertime, and the local public health department decides to use a gold standard test to test for step. This is usually a throat culture that is time-consuming and a bit expensive, and it shows that about 25% of all schoolchildren with sore throats in fact have strep. That means that out of 100 children with sore throat, 25 will have the potentially dangerous streptococcus organism as the cause. The doctor and the patient (and the parents!) don't want to wait two or three days for a throat culture result to come back from the laboratory to get confirmation; thus, the doctor has the following four situations to deal with:

1. The test can be positive and the organism is in fact present (a "true positive").
2. The test can be positive, but the organism is in fact not present (a "false positive").
3. The test can be negative, but the organism is actually present (that is, the test missed the organism, also called a "false negative").
4. The test can be negative and the organism is, in fact, not present (a "true negative").

We know that the streptozyme test that misses 5% or so of streptococcus cases and overdiagnoses 15% of sore throats as being due to strep when they are not. For 100 children, we would expect the results of their 100 streptozyme tests to look like Figure 5-2, if 25% of all of them in fact have strep (if they were all to have a time-consuming throat culture done).

So, how to interpret this? By looking at the chart, it's easy (and most physicians have software on their PDAs to do exactly this but they almost never use it). We can conclude the following from this chart.

First, if the streptozyme test is positive, only 25 of those 35 kids actually have strep; the other 11 kids show up as false positives. That means that there's about a 70% chance (25 divided by 35) that, if the test is positive, it is in fact due to strep—and, of course, a 30% chance that the test is wrong. But 70% makes for pretty high odds, and most reasonable physicians and parents would opt to treat their child for strep throat based on this information.

FIGURE 5-2. The results of a test for strep in 100 schoolchildren.

	Strep Present	Strep Absent	Total Test results positive or Negative
Test Positive	24	11	35
Test Negative	1	64	65
Total Strep Positive or Negative	25	75	

Second, if the streptozyme test is negative, since 65 out of 100 tests will be negative and 64 of those 65 test are true negatives, then there is about a 99% chance (64 divided by 65) that there is no strep. This is a very reassuring result!

Think of it this way: it's inaccurate for your physician to say that "you have strep" if the streptozyme test is positive. After all, there's only a 7 out of 10 chance that you do. But that's good enough for most people, especially since the treatment (with penicillin or a substitute drug for those allergic to penicillin) is inexpensive and doesn't carry much risk. And, in this case, if the test is negative, strep is—for all intents and purposes—ruled out.

A general statement can now be made about most screening tests: when uncertainty of the existence of a given malady is high—that is, we can't rule it in or out based on the physical examination alone—screening tests can help a lot.

GOOD TEST, BAD TEST: SAME TEST

But what if the condition is unlikely to exist in the first place? For example, in the summer—as opposed to the winter—strep is very rarely the cause of sore throats. Sore throats in summer are more likely to be due to a viral infection, which isn't treatable with antibiotics. Would a competent doctor use the streptozyme test to evaluate a patient with a sore throat in August? We can recalculate the same chart with the assumption that only 5% of 100 sore throats are actually due to strep, and the result looks like the chart in Figure 5-3.

The Meaning of a Positive and Negative Test Change
If the streptozyme test is positive, since there will be 19 positives out of any 100 sore throat patients tested, 15 of which will be false positives, the likelihood that strep is actually present is only 26% (4 in 19). Is that sufficient reason to treat? Many people would say no.

If the streptozyme test is negative, since 81 tests out of 100 sore

FIGURE 5-3. The results of a test when the strep is unlikely to exist in the first place.

	Strep Present	Strep Absent	Total Test results positive or Negative
Test Positive	4	15	19
Test Negative	1	80	81
Total Strep Positive or Negative	5	95	

throat patients will be negative, the probability of strep actually being absent is 99% (80 divided by 81).

So, even though the test is the same, the meaning of the result is different in summer versus winter. A positive test doesn't help very much, and a negative test result doesn't change the pretest likelihood of strep being absent (it was already 95% likely to be absent and testing increased that by a mere 4% or so).

A second general statement can now be made about most screening tests. If one has a high confidence of either the presence or absence of a given disease before the test is done, screening tests *don't help very much*. A more invasive—and thus potentially dangerous—test is necessary if there is really a need to know with near absolute confidence (such as in the case of some cancers).

Unfortunately, if you ask most doctors what the meaning of a positive streptozyme test is in the summer versus winter, the answer you'll get is "the same." That's wrong, and it can lead to deadly consequences, such as a fatal reaction to an antibiotic that wasn't needed in the first place.

THE POPULARITY OF SCREENING— UNCLE IVAN AND THE CT SCAN

For a more consequential example, suppose you want to know if you have coronary artery disease, even though you have no symptoms. Set aside the issue of whether we can do much to reverse early coronary disease other than what mom taught you about eating right and exercising. Perhaps your concern is that a distant uncle in Russia died from a heart attack at the age of 59, which happens to be your age. What might a doctor do? What might he or she tell you?

It turns out it that the answer depends on which doctor you ask—which isn't very reassuring. All doctors should know about coronary disease since it is so common in the United States, and that means they should be familiar with screening tests for coronary disease. Let's say you happen to get lucky and wind up seeing a thoughtful physician. She will determine that your blood pressure is normal, that you don't smoke, that your cholesterol is fine, and that, aside from Uncle Ivan (and who knows what life was doing to him in Russia?), there is no other family history of heart disease.

She elicits with a careful history that you play tennis six times a week without chest pain or undue shortness of breath and that you sweat when it is hot outside during your games, but otherwise feel fine. From this information alone—that is, based just on talking with you—your smart doctor knows that your chances of coronary disease are, at most, 1% or 2%. She reassures you and advises that you come back for another physical exam in five years.

But you're not happy. You want to be *absolutely* certain that you don't end up like Uncle Ivan. So you demand a stress test, where you are put on a treadmill while your heart rate and electrocardiogram (which shows the flow of electricity in the heart) are measured. Your doctor counsels against it, saying that (just like the streptozyme test), "It is far from a perfect test. And, besides, you are doing a stress test six times a week with your tennis games and you haven't fallen over dead yet."

Indeed, the formal exercise stress test has a false positive rate of at least 15%, and, since your chances of coronary disease are only 1%, a "positive" stress test is 15 times more likely to be inaccurate than accurate. Or think of it this way: 14 out of 15 times a positive stress test is a false positive in situations like the one described here, meaning that there is only about a 7% chance that, even if your stress test is positive, you actually have serious coronary disease.

You insist anyway. A good doctor would tell you to find another doctor, but let's say your physician is trying to be nice, so she orders the stress test. And let's say it comes back positive. Now what?

Depending on your willingness to live with uncertainty, you might ask to see a cardiologist. Fine, says your doctor, who's now grateful that you're going to be somebody else's problem. She refers you to "the best cardiologist in town." This cardiologist has an advanced CT scanner in his office (which he bought for $2 million) that can detect calcium in the coronary arteries, and he'll tell you that everybody with coronary artery atherosclerosis (which is hard to see on CT scan) has calcium deposits in their coronary arteries (and calcium shows up readily on a CT scan).

What he doesn't tell you is that one out of every five people your age *also* have coronary calcium deposits, and most of those 20% of folks do *not* have atherosclerosis. That's because calcium deposits are a normal aging phenomenon and do not in and of themselves constitute a "disease" that needs to be treated.

So you slap down a fat check for $300 for your coronary CT scan. Why? Most insurance companies won't pay for it. Sure enough, there are calcium deposits in "minimal to moderate" concentration in your coronary arteries. The cardiologist—if he is being honest (and so far he hasn't been)—will tell you that your chances of having narrowed coronary arteries is "low." By "low," he means less than 5% to 10%, not much different from what you already knew after the stress test. Feeling better now?

Probably not. So you opt for the only test that can definitively resolve the uncertainty in your mind: a cardiac catheterization. Financial considerations aside ($2,000 for the cardiologist performing it, about twice that much for the use of the catheterization suite), this test is invasive in the extreme. Small catheters are threaded up your arm or leg all the way to the heart. The tip of the catheter is inserted directly into the coronary arteries, and dye is squirted in under high pressure. (Perhaps not exactly what the arteries were designed to accommodate.) The test is, by definition, the gold standard. However, just *doing* the test subjects you to a risk of about one chance in 1,000 of dying. Add to that one chance in 200 of bleeding or nonfatal heart damage requiring hospitalization. That's probably greater than your chance of dying from coronary disease in the first place!

The test is performed, and you have no adverse effects except for a very sore leg and two weeks of no tennis to give your arterial puncture wound time to heal. You also have no coronary disease seen.

Was it worth it? It's hard to say in an individual case, but from numerous studies we know that, on a population basis, the answer is no. Far too many unneeded catheterizations are done—some because doctors don't know how to do the simple arithmetic just described and some because they have a very strong financial incentive to do so. Bottom line: in 2002 about 1.3 million cardiac catheterizations were performed at a cost of more than $6,000 each. That's about $10 billion, or roughly 1% of the entire health care budget in the United States for one procedure.

To be fair, if you had reported to your doctor that you had chest pain every time you climbed a single flight of stairs, that you smoked a pack of cigarettes a day, that your 62-year-old brother had a heart attack at age 55, and that both of your parents died from coronary artery disease, no stress test would be necessary (nor would the fancy CT scan looking for coronary calcium). It would be straight to the catheterization lab for you, with a view toward fixing the blockages that would inevitably be present.

TERRORIZED BY TECHNOLOGY

Pick up almost any newspaper in a major metropolitan area, and you'll find an advertisement or two on the latest scanning technology that can give you peace of mind for a piece of your wallet. MRI and CT scans are now ubiquitous and can image the blood vessels in your coronary arteries, look for unusual spots in your lungs where cancer might occur, detect unusual spots in your liver where cancer might be hiding, and then lead to further invasive tests.

These total body scans are, from a scientific standpoint, the epitome of malpractice. There is not only no evidence that they increase the quantity or quality of life, but there is extraordinary evidence that they increase anxiety, not to mention the costs and number of follow-on invasive procedures, each of which, of course, has an associated risk. Now the minimal good news here is that there are—at long last—a few prospective control trials looking at the benefits of total body scanning for the early detection of cancer in high-risk populations such as smokers, and for the early detection of coronary disease in high-risk patients, such as those with hypertension or bad family histories.

But the results are not yet in. If past is prologue—and there is virtually no exception to this lesson so far—it is highly likely that these new technologies, widely applied, will lead to far more mortality and morbidity than they save. That is in distinction to having a scan if one is symptomatic. For example, a smoker with a chronic cough (but *not* all smokers per se) *may* benefit from having a scan of their lungs to look for the presence of early lung cancer, although our track record in discovering early lung cancer, operating on it, or treating it with chemotherapy is not promising. Even in the symptomatic smoker, there is as yet no evidence that early detection of lung cancer means longer survival; indeed, it may mean both shorter survival and a lower quality of life due, for example, a surgical procedure to remove a large portion of the lungs in the hope of keeping the cancer from spreading. Despite the "common sense" nature of the attempt, biology is rarely as simple as that.

It may well be that one day we will have new techniques for treating early cancer that will make the discovery of early cancer beneficial. But that hope aside, the use of body scanning or heart scanning is a marketing ploy done by physicians for the sole purpose of making money and leveraging the anxiety or the fear and dread of the unknown. Tests like these—sophisticated and attractive as the advertisements are—should be avoided.

This is not an isolated or unsubstantiated view. Both the American Radiology Association and the American Academy of Cardiologists have stated in multiple position papers and guidelines for physicians that all of these scanning tests should be considered experimental and inherently dangerous outside of controlled trials. If one wishes to enroll in a controlled trial where one is randomized to either receive a total body scan or not and then to measure actual health outcome sometime down the line—2, 5, or 10 years—that is ethically acceptable, but subjects should not have to pay for the research.

Ruling out the presence of disease has an enticing, hypnotic appeal with an as yet unproven promise of increasing the quality and quantity of your life. Despite more than a decade's worth of experience of heart scans and total body scans in asymptomatic individuals who are looking to remain healthy, there has been no demonstrable benefit whatsoever from their use. Rather, the incidence of false positive results, which begins the diagnostic cascade of ever more invasive tests, leads not only to increased costs but to risk to life itself.

SCREENING GONE AWRY

A plethora of other screening tests have come onto the medical market in the past decade, and almost all have disappeared as fast they grabbed headlines as the next great "preventive" test. Perhaps people at risk for certain diseases pressured their physicians into using the tests, believing that they would benefit. Perhaps physicians themselves felt that if they didn't do the new screening test they might be subject to a malpractice lawsuit if the patient turned out to have the disease the test was supposed to detect. And perhaps on occasion the physician invested in a laboratory or radiology facility that did the test and hoped to make a profit by utilizing the screening procedure on as many patients as possible.

Consider the case of a 65-year-old cigarette smoker who has an annual physical examination. The doctor finds nothing specific upon examination and the only complaint the patient has is a chronic cough. In addition, the patient gets short of breath with minimal exercise, probably due to emphysema from 40 years of smoking two packs of cigarettes a day.

The doctor has read about a "new, exciting" screening test called a "multichannel chest CT" that can find lesions or growths in the lung as small as 2 millimeters (less than a tenth of an inch) in diameter, and he orders the test to make sure the patient doesn't have cancer.

The CT scan result shows a small mass in the periphery of one lung (possibly a cancer, possibly not); so the patient is referred to a pulmonary surgeon. The surgeon does a biopsy of the growth, which shows a type of cancer called "adenocarcinoma." This type of cancer has an average survival of five years, meaning 50% of patients with this condition will be dead after five years, and 50% will still be alive. The surgeon recommends that the patient have the growth removed, a procedure that involves the removal of an entire lobe of the already poorly functioning lung. But, because the surgery is very invasive and because the patient has emphysema, he does not survive the operation. Thus, the screening test led to a bad result. Figure 5-4 illustrates the flow of events and the unfortunate outcome.

But there's something else that needs to be considered: if the surgeon or primary doctor had thought about it, this patient had a bad prognosis to start off with because of his emphysema. He probably wouldn't have lived five years anyway. So the screening test took an already bad situation—an expected longevity of five years due to the

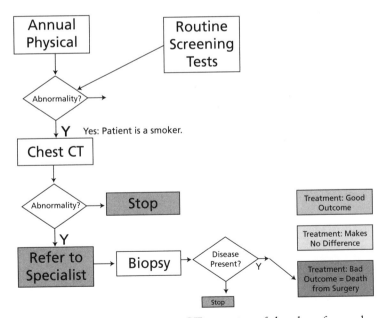

FIGURE 5-4. Screening gone awry—CT scanning of the chest for smokers to detect cancer.

emphysema—and made it worse by subjecting the patient to a danger-ous procedure that in this case was fatal, even though the screening test was very "sensitive": it identified the probable cancer but it didn't matter. The patient died *with* his cancer and not *because* of it.

The lesson here for physicians is that it is not enough to identify disease early; it is critical to know if something useful can be done about it, what difference the treatment makes, and what risks are asso-ciated with the treatment. This kind of lesson is learned very slowly by individual physicians and throughout the health care industry. The process of analysis that leads to the best possible conclusion (not nec-essarily the conclusion one wants to hear, but the scientifically credi-ble one) is called "systems analysis," and it has been practiced in engineering and science fields for many decades. Only recently has it come to medicine, largely because the vast majority of physicians are not trained to think as scientists and even fewer have learned the rela-tively simple mathematics needed to do the analysis.

The lesson for patients is to always ask a question of themselves and their physicians: what difference will a given screening test make to the quality and quantity of my life?

Diagnostic tests—screening tests included—are useful only when:

- There is a truly ambiguous knowledge of whether a given con-dition exists—say, a confidence of 20% to 80%, despite a good history and an exam expertly performed by a doctor.

- Early detection makes a difference in treating a disease.

- The potential for harm from starting down a wild goose chase with multiple tests is small.

- The test itself has limited risk.

- The disease that the test is designed to detect can, in fact, be treated with a high percentage of success or cured.

- The treatment of the disease doesn't result, on average, in side effects that are as bad as (or worse than) as the disease itself.

Thinking about this isn't an option. It is imperative. Unfortu-nately, most physicians don't.

PITFALLS AND PROMISES IN CANCER SCREENING TESTS

Like most patients, physicians assume that the more information they have about an individual or a specific problem, the better the outcome will be. For example, if a patient has long-standing heart disease, it would seem to be just common sense that an extra EKG, a stress test every year, or maybe one of the new (and expensive) non-invasive MRI-imaging scans, which show whether there are new obstructions in the coronary arteries, would be desirable tests to perform. We have seen that that is rarely the case and that, in fact, more information leads to more opportunity for misinterpretation and then poor decision making on therapies that in and of themselves pose danger. Like it or not, the biology of diseases can rarely be parsed by reason and logic because it is so terribly complex. The law of unintended consequences applies routinely, certainly much more than most physicians are taught in their training.

There is also a belief that screening tests—because they detect disease earlier than it might otherwise manifest itself—almost always lead to better outcomes. What could be bad about discovering a disease of any kind in its earliest stages? Attractive as this logic seems, only a few screening tests have turned out to be beneficial, and many more have turned out to actually be harmful.

LENGTH- AND LEAD-TIME BIAS

Two of the inherent problems with screening tests are not completely obvious to patients, but they should be well understood by doctors. Regrettably, they are not. There are "biases"—distortions in the meaning of the information—built into just about all screening tests to a minor or major degree.[1]

Assuming screening tests are utilized when the correct conditions, as just listed, are met, can they still result in more harm than good? The answer is yes, and it's due not to the tests themselves, but to the very nature of disease. If you think that physicians have difficulty with the core concepts of diagnostic testing, such as sensitivity and specificity, they tend to know even less about the inherent fallacies of screening tests called "lead time" and "length time" bias.

Lead time bias means that a screening test can *appear* to result in improvements in life expectancy but don't because the disease they are designed to detect typically don't cause any problems early on in their course. Let's consider the early diagnosis of breast cancer using mammography.

The most common form of breast cancer begins as a small collection of cells in the milk ducts of the female breast (and very, very rarely in male breast tissue as well). These cells are actively dividing all the time, and so occasionally errors are made when the DNA of the cells is copied, leading to cells that grow more quickly than they should and often don't stay put where they are supposed to be—the very definition of cancer. As long as the abnormal cells remain localized in a small region in the milk ducts of the breast, they are harmless. It's when the collection of cells gets large enough to grow beyond the ducts *or* when for some reason a cell or two detach from their abnormal cousins and manage to find their way into the bloodstream that the trouble starts—a metastasis. In breast cancer (but not necessarily in other cancers), it is almost always the case that the more abnormal cells that are present, the greater the likelihood is for a metastasis to take place. Thus, cancer specialists postulated many years ago, based on very intense study of the basic biology and behavior of breast cancer cells, that early detection and removal of the tiniest growths would make a positive difference in outcomes, preventing either metastasis or very disfiguring breast masses that could be difficult to deal with even if none of the cells successfully metastasized elsewhere.

It is helpful to understand that when cancer cells break off from the original site of growth—called the "primary" site by oncologists—they don't end up in random places in the body. Primary cancers in a given organ have well described propensities to lodge themselves in other specific organs when they metastasize. Breast cancer cells that get into the bloodstream don't survive to cause serious problems unless they end up in other organs that, for very complex reasons that are far from completely understood, support their growth. Indeed, it is the rule that the primary cancer site is almost never the reason for the death of a cancer patient. It is the *metastatic* sites—where cells from one organ take up residence in another organ and destroy the function of the *secondary* organ that is often responsible for an individual's demise.

Breast cancer cells are, unfortunately, among the least choosy of the other organs in which they will take up residence, probably because the cells can secrete chemical substances that will stimulate the growth of new blood supply—literally to feed the metastasis—just about anywhere. Thus, the most common metastatic sites of breast cancer are bones, the lungs, the liver, and the brain. Occasionally breast cancer will metastasize to the ovaries, to the adrenal glands (which make a wide variety of absolutely essential hormones necessary for the health of organs everywhere in the body and thus the body as whole), and even to the opposite breast.

So it's rather easy to predict what will happen as a result of these metastases from breast cancer: if a bone is the new host site—perhaps a vertebra in the back or the femur or pelvic bones—the bone will become weakened and may fracture even with normal use. These are called "pathological fractures" because they occur not as a result of trauma forces exceeding the capacity of the bones to maintain their structure, but rather as a result of severe damage to the very structure of the bones themselves. Pathological fractures are not only extremely painful, but fixing the fracture can be very difficult, if not impossible. It is necessary, of course, to kill the cancer cells themselves—usually done with radiation therapy and sometimes with chemotherapy—and then surgically repairing the fracture site. Since radiation inhibits healing, surgically repaired pathological fractures may remain unstable—and terribly painful—for many months.

Metastasis to the lung can cause a myriad of problems. If the unwelcome breast cancer cells block airway passages—that is, the bronchial tubes—normal secretions can't be cleared out by coughing, and bacteria can grow unimpeded: a pneumonia, or what physicians call a "postobstructive pneumonia." Antibiotics may not be adequate to clear the infection. Once again, the breast cancer cells have to be killed with either radiation or chemotherapy, but both of these modalities impede the function of the immune system, which acts in concert with antibiotics to destroy the bacteria. If the immune system is functioning poorly, even in just a small area such as the portion of the lung that has been irradiated, antibiotics are much less effective and sometimes not effective at all. Infection is thus a common final cause of death in patients with breast cancer, even in the modern era when there are dozens of powerful antibiotics to choose from.

Similarly, if breast cancer metastasizes to the liver, it can grow so prolifically as to replace the normal liver cells—responsible for clearing toxins from the bloodstream and for manufacturing essential proteins. Without these proteins—for example, albumin, the primary protein in the blood serum—numerous functions throughout the body go away.

Finally, many cancers—breast cancer included—can suppress appetite. Just about all readers know someone who has had cancer of one primary type or another who lose much weight during treatment or before death. The cancer cells produce a variety of materials that have been shown to cause chronic nausea and undermine the body's natural sensors that drive appetite (located in the brain and stomach). Poor nutrition alone can result in death from cancer.

These are the effects of cancer that we seek to avoid with screening. If a new tumor can be literally "nipped in the bud" before it metastasizes, all of these horrible effects—most of them ultimately fatal—can be obviated. In the specific case of breast cancer, we have been able to prove that early detection works most of the time. The routine use of mammography to find early breast cancer has saved many lives and spared much suffering. But it doesn't always work, and, oddly enough, attempts to improve on standard mammography to find even smaller tumors or tumors that are hard to visualize with ordinary X-rays haven't led to the improvements in survival that were first realized about 20 years ago. Let's explore this a bit more.

In brief, the success of mammography derives from the fundamental behavior of *most* early breast cancers. From many years of careful laboratory research, we know that from the start of breast cancer until a 1-centimeter ball of cells is formed (roughly the size that a woman can feel with monthly self-exam), the development takes about five or six years. Most—but not all—of the time, the breast lump is confined to the breast in this situation and can be removed and treated with local radiation and (relatively) mild chemotherapy, and the treatment results in greater than a 90% cure. Since a woman who has survived breast cancer is obviously at higher-than-average risk for a second breast cancer, continued follow-up mammograms and self-examination are necessarily indefinitely. But the process works and works well.

However, there are powerful lessons for other screening tests from those few women who go on to die from breast cancer *despite* early detection. We'll postulate that, in a given patient, the rare aggressive breast cancer lasts for something less than six years before killing the individual. If the women detects it by palpation at, perhaps, three years into the course of the cancer and then dies three years later, we would conclude that the disease is fatal in three years (six minus three), or we might say that "the median survival with this cancer is three years." If, on the other hand, the mammogram detects the cancer two years before—when it is very small but growing aggressively—and the patient dies five years later (because the therapy doesn't work), we would say that "the median survival with this cancer is five years." So, even though it is exactly the same cancer—with the same unfortunate result—the screening test appears to have improved survival by two years simply because the patient had a two-year "lead time" in detecting it. Put another way, the screening test artificially increased the apparent survival from this particular type of aggressive breast cancer. In reality, nothing changed because this unusual, particularly aggressive cancer was going to be fatal no matter what physicians tried to do. Finding it early only appeared to improve survival; hence the phrase "lead-time bias," an artifact of finding an otherwise fatal disease earlier than it would be found by waiting until a lump could be felt by the patient or some other effect of metastatic disease became apparent.

So, to put it simply, "lead-time bias" means that the screening tests give a false impression of prolonging survival. If one detects a disease that is very aggressive and that will result in death no matter what is done or not done, knowing about it early doesn't help. It *seems* to help only because patients know earlier than they otherwise would. Thus the person is alive longer with *the knowledge of having the disease* but the screening test did not, in fact, prolong life because no treatment can alter the course of certain aggressive diseases. Fortunately, this is not usually the case with breast cancer, but it is, for example, the case with pancreatic cancer. We don't have any good screening tests for pancreatic cancer, but, even if we did, early detection probably would make no difference because it tends to metastasize quite early in the course of the disease. Patients would know—regrettably for longer than they otherwise would have—that they were living with a disease that would probably kill them and that little could be done about it.

A second type of screening test bias is called *length-time bias* and is in some ways the opposite of lead-time bias. In this case, a screening test turns up an abnormal growth that is so slow growing that it never would have caused a problem in the first place. The classic example of length-time bias is in the use of the PSA test for prostate cancer. To see why, one has to understand a bit about normal prostate physiology and the tendency of the prostate cells to gradually change with age—sometimes so much that, if some of these cells are harvested with a biopsy, they look like they *might* be cancer.

TESTING FOR PROSTATE CANCER

The prostate gland—a walnut-sized organ wedged between the base of the male bladder and the colon—gradually enlarges in almost all men as they get older. Since the urethra (the tube that carries urine out of the bladder to the penis for elimination) passes directly through the substance of the prostate, it can literally get squeezed by the surrounding prostate tissue, thus accounting for the slow urination and sense of an "incomplete" bladder emptying that many men start to experience in their fifties and sixties. It's a virtually universal phenomenon by the age of seventy, and it has nothing to do with prostate cancer per se. To look at a little differently, prostate cancer is almost never the cause of the urinary symptoms that men experience as they age. As long as prostate cancer remains in the prostate gland, it virtually never causes symptoms.

As the prostate grows with age—a biologic curiosity called "*benign prostatic hypertrophy*" (BPH)—the cells of the bladder secrete into the bloodstream more and more of a protein product called the "prostate specific antigen" (PSA). So, PSA levels—easily detectable with a simple blood test—tend to slowly rise with age.

About 25 years ago it was recognized that prostate *cancer* cells, because they are growing more quickly than normal prostate cells, secrete *more* PSA into the bloodstream. A bright researcher got the idea then that, if the PSA was elevated above the normal range, it might be an indicator of cancer cells in the prostate. And it turned out that the researcher was correct.

It is important to understand that, unlike breast cancer, prostate cancer is *very* slow growing in most men who have it. In fact, we now know that by age 65, about a third of men who die from unrelated causes and have an autopsy done have abnormal prostate cells—which pathologists classify as cancer—in their prostate glands, as Figure 5-5 shows.

Notice that the figure shows two curves: one for latent cancer, which is defined as cancer found incidentally at autopsy, and one for clinical prostate cancer, which means cancer detected while a male patient is alive. Almost always the detection takes place because the PSA is elevated, and this finding then leads to a prostate biopsy that reveals the abnormal cells.

But herein lies a serious problem with the screening test. Since so many men (most, in fact, by age 70) have, in their prostate glands, abnormal cells that we *call* cancer, but since most men make it to age 70 *without* their prostate cancer cells metastasizing or otherwise causing any noticeable trouble of any kind, *who* among the many millions of men with elevated PSA blood levels will, in fact, need to have a procedure to remove (or irradiate) their prostate glands so that they won't suffer the effects of metastatic disease? The answer is that we simply do not know.

Over the years, pathologists have attempted to "score" the degree of abnormality of prostate cancer cells based on the size of the chromosome (or DNA) in the cells because their experience with other cancers extra or extra-large DNA often indicates that the cell has a propensity to metastasize. In addition, pathologists try to look at the pattern of the prostate cells under the microscope to see if the organi-

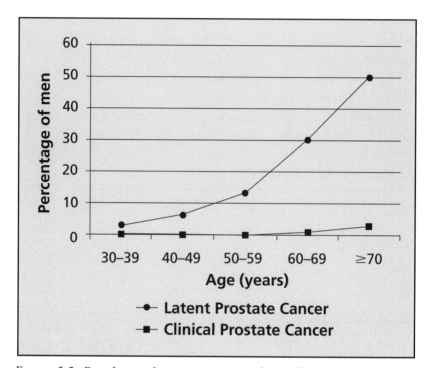

FIGURE 5-5. Prevalence of prostate cancer with age (from G. P. Hass, et al. "The Role of Prevalence in the Diagnosis of Prostate Cancer," *Cancer Control* 13;3: 158–167.

zation of the cells gives any hint as to whether the cells are sticking close together—as they normally do—or are coming apart, perhaps an early indicator of a propensity to metastasize.

This "scoring" or "grading," of the prostate cells was first attributed to Dr. Donald Gleason in 1977 and thus came to be known as the Gleason Score, and it is done by looking at two separate clusters of abnormal cells obtained at biopsy and assigning a number of 1 to 5 to each cluster, with 1 meaning normal cells and 5 meaning wildly abnormal cells. Obviously, the intervening numbers mean that the cells appear less ominous than the worst grade of 5.

This is not an easy assessment to make, and pathologists spend many months in their training looking at hundreds of prostate biopsies to learn how to differentiate among them. Schematically and also under the microscope, Figure 5-6 shows what some of the grades of prostate cancer cells look like; the differences can be rather subtle and are sometimes subject to a bit of judgment and guesswork.

To calculate the Gleason Score, the pathologist looks at two representative samples from biopsies of a patient's prostate gland. If the pathologist finds one cluster of cells that is Grade 3 and a second cluster that shows much disorganization and lots of DNA per cell with a Grade of 5, the total Gleason score is $5 + 3 = 8$. The maximum Gleason score is 10, and the lowest is 2.

There is no question that the Gleason score predicts who is most likely to *eventually* show evidence of metastasis of prostate cancer, and, since prostate cancer has a nasty tendency to spread to bone and lung (much like breast cancer does in females), it can cause a great deal of suffering. Further, since men with metastatic prostate cancer may live

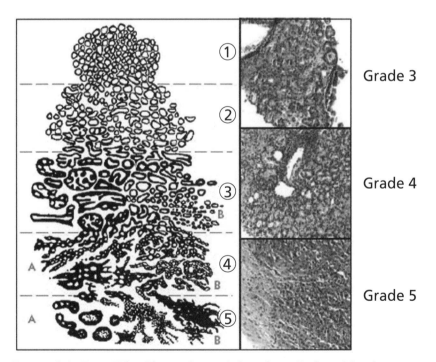

FIGURE 5-6. From "The Gleason Score: A Significant Biologic Manifestation of Prostate Cancer Aggressiveness on Biopsy." *Prostate Cancer Research Insights* 4(1), available on the Internet at http://www.prostate-cancer.org.

a long time because prostate cancer cells, even when metastatic, are slow growing, the suffering can be quite prolonged. As a former prostate cancer patient of one of the authors of this book used to say, "This is not a good way to die." He ultimately took his own life because of intractable pain. Unfortunately, despite the predictive value of the Gleason score, there is *no* evidence to date that if the urologist removes the prostate of a patient with a high Gleason score in the hope of preventing metastasis that it does any good. Why? The tumor *may have already metastasized* by the time the operation is done, but the cells are so tiny (and grow so slowly) that no CAT scanner or any other test can show where they may be hiding and waiting to cause problems. In short, the patient may undergo a painful, disfiguring procedure that also carries with it a high risk of impotence and urinary incontinence, yet the cancer may reappear two years later with a sudden pathological fracture and indescribable pain.

At the same time, if a patient has an elevated PSA and then undergoes a prostate biopsy where the Gleason score is toward the lower end of the scale (say 4), should the patient have the prostate removed? Most urologists will say yes, but there is no way to know that that particular patient will ever have any risk of metastasis. The patient may thus undergo the same radical prostate removal procedure—or high-dose radiation therapy—for naught. And, in the process of so doing, it will *appear* that the intervention "cured" the patient, when in reality the patient never would have had problems in the first place. This is called "length-time bias," a complicated way of saying that it just so happens that the screening test identified a group of patients—and perhaps a very large group of patients since most men who under prostate biopsy have total Gleason scores less than 7—who really didn't have disease that would actually shorten their lives. The length of time they would have lived would have been long in any case. So, instead of a true disease that could kill them, they had a mere pathological oddity when their biopsy sample was viewed under the microscope.

Thus, the length-time bias of the screening test for prostate cancer can—and, in fact, often does—create a terrible conundrum for the patient. We can most certainly detect the prostate cancer, we can give the patient a rough (sometimes very rough) idea of the likelihood of metastatic disease, but we can't say for sure that removing the prostate gland—which is the only way to be sure all of the localized prostate cancer is removed—removes the risk of metastatic disease. It may have already occurred. Nor can we tell the patient with a low Gleason score that he will *not* someday have metastatic disease. Even if the Gleason score is as low as possible (a value of "2"), the biopsy procedure may have *missed* the areas of the gland where prostate cancer cells with metastatic potential are reproducing.

What to do? With our current technology and understanding of the behavior of prostate cancer cells, the only proper approach is a controlled trial, essentially a study of two groups of men: those with known prostate cancer on biopsy who do *not* have treatment done and those with known prostate cancer who undergo a procedure in an attempt at a cure. At the moment, there are three treatment options: (1) radical prostatectomy, a long surgical procedure to remove the prostate gland that can damage nerves controlling bladder and erectile function; (2) implantation of tiny radioactive pellets (called "seeds") to destroy the prostate gland, which can cause radiation damage to nearby organs such as the colon and the bladder; (3) external radiation, which can also damage other organs. We then wait—years are necessary—to see if there is a difference in outcome. The European Randomized Study of Screening for Prostate Cancer is one such trial. Results are expected in about 2010 or 2011 and will tell us several things:

- How much difference in terms of quantity *and* quality of life the screening test makes.

- Whether or not there is an appropriate age cutoff for screening for prostate cancer. After all, most men who are 70 years old are going to die from something other than prostate cancer (such as heart disease or stroke, even though the majority have what appear to be" cancer cells in the prostate.

- Whether screening does more harm than good by creating a large cohort of men who have undergone a radical prostatectomy or radiation therapy and whose quality of life is so bad as to, perhaps, be not worth living, at least in the view of those men. Obviously different individuals will have different opinions on how bad life really is with, say, urinary incontinence as a result of radical prostatectomy, and we'll return to this key point—patient preference—several times in the remainder of this book.

Until the results of the European study are known, any male considering a PSA screening test should ask himself one very difficult question: "*Am I prepared to live with the result of the test?*" Or, to put it another way, if the test is positive, am I ready to undergo a prostate biopsy and act on the results of that test knowing that I may or may *not* be improving my longevity while I subject myself to the risk of unpleasant—and usually irreversible—side effects from the treatment? In our view, it is incumbent upon the physician who recommends a PSA screening test to a patient to have this discussion *before* the test is ordered.

Unfortunately, this is not common practice among family physicians, internists, or even urologists. Such a discussion is a long one because the answer to one question on something as potentially consequential as finding cancer leads to many others, and primary care physicians are already under much time pressure to see as many patients as possible in a day. Few insurance companies or patients themselves are willing to pay for the pretest counseling involved (even though such counseling, properly done, may save insurance companies money while at the same time sparing patients much suffering). It may also be the case that some physicians—urologists in particular—are disinterested in such a discussion because it may mean they have fewer chances to perform what is a very lucrative procedure. In addition, it is fair to say physicians aren't trained adequately in helping patients think through uncertainty, what researchers in the field of decision and analysis refer to as "assessment of disutility." This is easier to do when deciding among the various refrigerators to purchase than in medical therapy or screening choices, which tend to involve much more emotion and possible adverse consequences. And make no mis-

take: until the results of the European study are available (and con-
firmed by other studies that will report further into the future),
physicians and patients have to deal with a high degree of uncertainty
with the PSA screening test.

As is clear, lead- and length-time biases complicate immensely the
evaluation of various screening tests. But, as a result of gathering much
data over several decades we've been able to take these important—
and often overlooked—factors into account. We've learned that many
screening tests that seem to be beneficial aren't. Worse, if the screening test leads to a procedure that harms the patient but impacts the
underlying disease hardly at all, it is indeed worse than worthless.

Because the diagnosis of prostate cancer is made so commonly
today, additional aspects of its treatment—including the decision not
to treat—are covered in the next chapter as well.

Testing for Breast Cancer

In the cases of breast cancer and prostate cancer, we've seen two more
or less opposite lessons on the actual usefulness of screening tests.
Mammography has clearly resulted in fewer deaths among women—
and far less suffering as well—from breast cancer and metastatic breast
cancer. And there are at least three reasons for this: the test itself is
reasonably sensitive, that is, *if* a breast cancer is present, the standard
mammogram is very likely to identify it in a curable stage. Second,
even though the test generates false positives—that is, it is far less than
100% specific for identifying breast cancer and may incorrectly lead to
the impression that a shadow on the X-ray is breast cancer when it is
not—the consequences of this inherent weakness in the test aren't too
awful: a breast biopsy and maybe a lumpectomy that ultimately show
no cancer. The surgery isn't terribly disfiguring and the discomfort and
costs are manageable. Third, and at least as important as the first two
reasons, is that we have after much trial and error found an intervention *that actually works* for preventing breast cancer from changing
from a small ball of cells into a life-threatening disease. We now know
with a high degree of confidence that the combination of lumpectomy,
local (not systemic) radiation therapy, and *relatively mild* chemotherapy

(few cancer chemotherapies are pleasant) effects a cure in 90% of people.

One might also note that no other screening test has demonstrated superiority over mammography. We also know that it is *probably* the case—we actually don't know for sure—that most early breast cancers *will* progress to disease that can do real harm if they are not removed. Put another way, early detection via mammography, the removal of the breast cancer, and the use of radiation and chemotherapy to destroy the last remaining cells increase quantity and quality of life. Waiting until a breast cancer becomes metastatic before treating it almost never results in a good outcome for the patient (it is indeed striking how little improvement over the past 30 years there has been in longevity and quality of life in women with already metastasized breast cancer). On balance then, the costs and risks of breast cancer screening result in a net positive for women. Still, on occasion, an early breast cancer will have already metastasized when it is detected by mammography. In these patients, we've made few advances in improving quality or quantity of life.

With prostate cancer, the story is about the opposite from breast cancer as one can imagine. Our one commonly available screening test—the PSA test—is very non-specific so that, if it turns up positive (as it does in as many as 5% to 10% of men who decide to get the test) many men feel compelled to go to the next step—a prostate biopsy—which is quite uncomfortable—and where results are not nearly so definitive in predicting outcome or guiding treatment. Suffice it to say that until the European study results are available sometime between the time of the writing of this book and 2010 or so, we simply are guessing, but at least a group of thoughtful researchers is making an effort to do the necessary study.

WHAT MAKES SENSE?

Twenty years of real-world experience with many screening tests show that only a small handful make much difference. In family practice, where most screening tests are done, academic researchers have summarized the positive and negative lessons just illustrated with a short set of requirements for "successful screening." They have determined that key issues must be addressed before any type of screening is adopted on a wide scale in order to avoid doing more harm than good:

1. Is the question we are trying to resolve—for example, the presence or absence of a specific condition—clear?
2. Are alternative strategies other than screening clearly defined, along with the costs and benefits of those alternatives?
3. Has the effectiveness of the intervention been convincingly demonstrated?
4. Are future costs and benefits computed and appropriately discounted?
5. What is the range of actual cost effectiveness estimated?
6. Has the effectiveness of the screening test been duplicated in more than one study?

Of these items, what policy makers and individuals want to know is,: "What does it cost to prevent one case of a given disease using a particular screening method?" (Individuals, of course, don't care what it costs when it comes to any given person, and there's no way to put a price on a human life.) How does one do that?

For better or worse, the best expression of cost-effectiveness we have is cost per quality-adjusted life year saved (QALY). A quality-adjusted year of life is what statisticians mean by "a year of existence but with the irreversible effects of a stroke that leaves someone unable to speak or ambulate without assistance" or "a year of life but with limited activity due to chronic shortness of breath due to heart failure after a serious heart attack." So, if a normal year of life is given the value 1, the QALY of someone who survived a serious stroke might be 0.5 (or 50%), and for someone who survived a bad heart attack with a heart functioning at only 40% of normal might be 0.6. Indeed, some individuals would regard a year of life confined to bed, immobile and helpless and mute, to actually be not worth living at all. Over the years, a consensus has been reached for practically every common malady on how much the chronic effects of that malady reduces the value of life. (Of course, theologians will argue that any breath taken is a gift from Heaven, but that's another book.)

Similarly, when assessing the quality of life, one can take into account the adverse effects, if any, from a treatment to cure a patient of a disease. The removal of a breast cancer via a lumpectomy (removing the lump and not the whole breast) is minimally disfiguring in most cases. But removal of a prostate gland—which may result in impotence or permanent urinary incontinence—may significantly reduce the patient's quality of life (aside from the question of whether removing what appears to be prostate cancer makes any difference in most cases).

The U.S. Preventive Services (USPSTF) Task Force on screening tests, a body within U.S. Department of Health and Human Service's Agency for Healthcare Research and Quality, and a similar group in Canada have concluded that, among the many dozens of screening tests available, certain ones make economic sense. Figure 5-7 presents those tests, along with the diseases they are designed to detect or prevent, the cost per QALY, and the actual number of lives saved per year in the United States.

On the other end of the spectrum are the following screening tests are widely available (just look in your local newspaper or watch an evening's worth of commercials on television). They have either failed to have been shown to save lives—indeed, they may increase overall mortality in the people who receive them—or they may do so but only at enormous costs, for example, at the rate of millions of dollar for each year of life saved:

- Total body scanning with CT-X-ray or magnetic resonance imaging to look for cancer.

- Heart scanning to look for coronary disease (or coronary calcium as a marker for coronary narrowing).

- PSA testing for prostate cancer.

- Exercise stress testing in people without symptoms of heart disease (even in patients with family histories of coronary disease).

FIGURE 5-7. The U.S. Preventative Task Force on Screening Test chart.

Screening test	Disease targeted	Cost per QALY	Number of lives saved annually in US	Comments
Mammography (breast cancer)	Intraductal breast cancer (most common type of breast cancer)	$ 50,000	150,000	Recommended every one or two years in women over age 40
Pap smears	Cervical Cancer	$100,000	10,000	Reduces overall death rate by about 25%
Cholesterol	Coronary Artery Disease	$ 35,000	150,000	
Blood pressure	Stroke and Heart Disease	$ 32,000	200,000	
Colon cancer screening	Colon Cancer	$250,000	75,000	Using colonoscopy and taking into account deaths from perforation or other side effects
Bone density for women at age 65	Osteoporosis	$ 65,000		Mortality from hip fracture reduced by 20% over five years

- Chest X-rays or chest CT scanning in cigarette smokers (to look for lung cancer).

- Ultrasound of the pelvis (to look for ovarian cancer in women).

We do save lives with screening (following the recommendations of the USPSTF), and we also improve the quality of life at costs that most people would say are "reasonable." The caveat is that we don't have very many screening tests that actually do save lives, though don't expect the purveyor of the next miracle screening test to tell you that.

NOTE

1. We don't mean to imply in any way that new screening tests – or even new diagnostic tests – will always or even usually result in a bad result or unintended consequence. Rather, any new technology, screening test or drug that comes on to the market must be subjected to thorough controlled trials. While these take much time and are thus also expensive (and on extremely rare occasions delay the introduction of some important product or therapy), from the dozens of medications and tests that were thought to be breakthroughs but turned out to be worse-than-worthless in just the past decade, it is far more likely than not that prudence and careful, lengthy clinical trials are the only way we currently have of separating the beneficial from the harmful. Someday, fundamental understanding of inexplicably complex biological processes may help us to shortcut this tedious sounding process. For the moment, we have nothing better.

CHAPTER 6

News from the Front: The War on Prostate and Other Cancers

WHEN PRESIDENT RICHARD NIXON declared the War on Cancer in a famous speech[1] in 1971, the promise of success against cancer—specifically cancer that had already spread or metastasized—seemed to be right around the corner. At the time, more than 35 years ago, there had been reason for optimism. By lucky observation in the 1940s, it was discovered that sulfur mustard—developed exclusively as a chemical weapons agent (though never used) during World War II—could be used to treat certain forms of cancer of the lymph nodes (called "lymphoma"). Surgeons had developed techniques for removing localized cancers that had not yet spread. And, early use of primitive radiation therapy machines shrank tumors that had already spread to other organs. But hype and hope dominated; careful statistical analysis did not. So it was only with an intensive retrospective look at the poorly kept data that it became apparent that—aside from very occasional dramatic cures—killing cancer cells with chemotherapy or radiation had its limitations. "Chasing cancer with a knife"—a favorite phrase of surgeons—was, in general, recognized as impossible. Rather, each of these modalities would help to temporarily relieve the local symptoms of cancer growth—pressure or obstruction on a bronchial tube or perhaps the tumor growing in a vertebra causing excruciatingly painful symptoms—but they did little for overall survival time and quality of life.

More than 30 years and trillions of dollars later, just how well have we done? The answer, in general, is not very well. Despite the good intentions of doctors and nurses, especially those in the specialty of oncology (cancer therapeutics) the bulk of the limited success against cancer remains in the realm of early detection—that is, identifying and removing a cancer *before* it has metastasized. Since 1971, a small percentage of childhood cancers (some leukemias and lymphomas), metastatic testicular cancer, and some forms of breast cancer have succumbed to advances in chemotherapy and radiation therapy (typically combined). The problem is that these now curable cancers represent a tiny fraction of all metastatic cancers.[2] The truth is that the vast majority of cancers—once spread—remain incurable despite the availability of many dozens of new chemotherapeutic drugs and even the use of antibodies directed against cancer cells.

Prostate cancer in men and breast cancer in women alone account for nearly 40% of all cancer diagnoses during life (other cancers may be found at the autopsy table as asymptomatic, or "symptomless," findings). Colon cancer, the next most common cancer in both sexes, is only 25% as common as either prostate or breast cancer. If you're not much for math, that means that, over the course of your life, there's a little less than one in four or five chance that you'll get prostate cancer (if you're a man) or breast cancer (if you're a woman).

Again, we stress that this is an *average*. Averages are by their nature made up of higher and lower numbers. Therefore, these odds lump in the health enthusiast who religiously avoids cancer-causing substances and bad habits along with the dietary-challenged heavy smokers with a history of cancer in the family. Statistics tell you the overall picture, but they are not necessarily an individual's destiny; so, while it is true that on average we're about as likely as not to hear the word "cancer" from our health care providers during our lifetimes, there are clearly genetic and lifestyle factors that change the probability. And, of course, if you die of something else, such as coronary disease, you don't live long enough to get cancer because most forms of it are associated with aging.

In the United States, all things being equal, an adult can expect a 50% chance of developing *some* type of cancer in his or her lifetime. It's a little frightening to contemplate, but, over the course of a life-time, it all comes down to exactly the same odds as a flip of the coin. Heads, you're clear. Tails, well, that's part of what this chapter is about. Death is inevitable from *something*, of course, but what physicians find with diagnostic tests and call *"disease"* may very well not be disease at all. And, if the nondisease is thought to require treatment, the inevita-ble side effects of that therapy may reduce the quality and quantity of life. In this chapter, we focus on cancer, specifically on the most com-mon cancer in males—prostate cancer. We note the apparent acceler-ation in its diagnosis or prevalence in the past decade, and we tell you what we have learned. The lessons are sobering, not at all what physi-cians expected based on the standard teaching in medical school.

Like most lay individuals, when physicians or medical students learn that someone has cancer, they immediately want to spring into action. After all, for the most part, cancer if not removed will inevita-bly spread from where it started to other organs, perhaps many organs. Once spread, it will eventually kill the patient, either because of dam-aging effects on the organs to which it has spread or because the cancer secretes substances that interfere with multiple functions of the body: everything from appetite and a general sense of wellness to inhibiting other cell types from doing critical functions. Young physicians are taught that, if caught early enough, some cancers can be cured or at least dramatically slowed in their progress. They are also taught that doing nothing almost guarantees that the patient will suffer and that doing something outweighs doing nothing.

But prostate cancer breaks all these rules, and it is a clear lesson

in the importance of knowing what it is that you *don't* know before
acting.

HOW CANCERS CAUSE PROBLEMS

Prostate cancer, much like breast cancer in the 1970s to the present,
is perhaps the most instructive example of the progress and frustrations
in the treatment of *neoplastic*—"new growth"—disease. Like just about
all cancers, in its site of origin—that is, in the organ where it started—
the cancer cells are neither threatening nor problematic. For example,
colon cancer almost never grows so large within the colon itself as to
cause obstruction or even localized pain. Rather, the trouble begins
when cancer cells spread through the bloodstream or the lymph nodes
to other organs, interfering with the function of the organs as a whole
via, at least in part, co-opting some of the blood supply and nutrients.
Stomach cancer is much the same, though there are exceptions to this
otherwise good rule of thumb: for some rare cancers, such as ones that
originate in the brain or pancreas, the growth of new cells can literally
squeeze out normal cells in a particularly critical region of anatomical
real estate. This condition can cause seizures in the brain and obstruction of the tiny duct that carries pancreatic enzymes into the intestine,
which are necessary for the digestion of food. In some (but not most)
types of lung cancer that begin in one of the myriad of branches of the
bronchial tubes, the same type of condition may result from airway
obstruction.

But when "foreign" cells spread through the bloodstream or the
delicate lymphatic system and take up residence in tissues that are not
part of their organs of origin—the process called "mestatasizing"—
they often interfere with the function of the organ, though it almost
always takes many months for this to happen. For example, prostate or
breast tissue that grows to a large size within the substance of the lung
may literally fill a bronchial tube supplying air to a large portion of the
lung much like cancer originating in the lung can. Not only is it then
impossible for that portion of the lung to absorb oxygen and expel
carbon dioxide into the bronchial tube, but normal secretions that are

cleared by coughing cannot get out of the lung. The resulting infection is usually called "postobstructive pneumonia," because the infection occurs behind the tumor growth in the bronchial tube.

In addition, the foreign cells steal blood flow and nutrients from the "host" organ; indeed, many cancers that have metastasized to other organs have the ability to induce the production of new blood vessel growth directly into the tumor mass, literally diverting blood flow from surrounding cells. And a catastrophic, sudden demise supervenes if the tumor cells should happen to start growing in a particularly vulnerable place, such as next to a blood vessel or a bronchial tube, eroding into those structures and causing uncontrolled bleeding.

Some tumors that are removed probably don't need to be removed in the first place, as we'll see with prostate cancer, and in some parts of the body the surgery is disfiguring, debilitating, or both. Chemotherapy and radiation, even when used judiciously by experts, almost always have at least temporary side effects. And a few people die from even the relatively low doses used after the removal of a primary tumor discovered by screening. It remains for the physician and patient to discuss the pluses and minuses of using our current therapeutic modalities for the treatment of most metastatic cancers. For some patients, the additional months of life when balanced against the time spent dealing with side effects may mean that doing nothing is as acceptable as doing everything.

As we've already seen, there is no question that with *some* screening procedures—breast and skin cancer being the leading example—that early detection clearly translates into longer and completely disease-free life, the combination of quantity and quality that each of us hopes for. But with prostate cancer, *the* most common cancer in males, the story is not so hopeful at this time.

A CLOSER LOOK AT CANCER: INCIDENCE AND IMPACT

The experience with prostate cancer captures many of the conundrums of screening—whom to screen, what to do if abnormal cells are found—and the problems of metastasis. We have diagnosed prostate cancer much more frequently in the past two decades than ever before as a result of the availability of new screening techniques. But what good have we done?

Prostate cancer incidence—that is, the number of cases per 100,000 of population per year—has shot up dramatically, as Figure 6-1 from the National Cancer Institute makes clear. Does this mean there is some new epidemic of prostate cancer? Probably not. What it means is that more people are being diagnosed with prostate cancer. The percentage of men who have prostate cancer has likely not changed, especially considering that most men eventually have it anyway, but more testing has revealed more *apparent* disease.

To assess the success of modern medicine's struggle to treat and cure cancer, the question we must ask is simply, "Of the top five cancers in men and the top five in women (see Figure 6-2), which comprise far more than 90% of all cancers diagnosed, have we seen any turnaround in the dismal mortality statistics from the pre-War-on-Cancer days?" What else can we learn? Careful readers will also be asking, "If we haven't exactly *cured* many cancers in the past 30 years, have we increased longevity in those with metastatic disease?"

Prostate cancer—by far the most common cancer in men—and breast cancer—by far the most common in females—provide most of the answer to these questions.

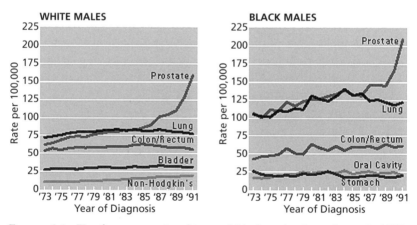

FIGURE 6-1. Top five cancers in white and black males from the early 1970s through the early 1990s. (Source: National Cancer Institute.)

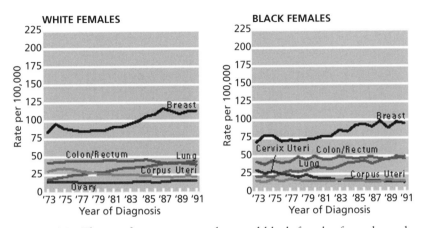

FIGURE 6-2. The top five cancers in white and black females from the early 1970s through the early 1990s. (Source: National Cancer Institute.)

THE RISE IN THE RATES OF PROSTATE CANCER

The data in Figure 6-1 is clear: There is an unmistakable increase in the incidence of prostate and breast cancer in the past few decades. There is general agreement that the increase in screening, per se, is at least partially responsible for the increase in these cancers. In other words, *since more people are being tested, more people are diagnosed.* Since mammography screening for breast cancer *slowly* became standard practice over the course of about at decade, it is unsurprising that the incidence of identified breast cancer rose at a similarly slow rate. For black women—generally poorer and with less access to medical care of all types—the rise in early breast cancer detection has been delayed because the use of mammography was simply less on average. We now recognize that black females have a chance of developing breast cancer that is about on par with white females.

Prostate cancer incidence, on the other hand, took a massive jump in the late 1980s and early 1990s with the arrival of the prostate-specific antigen (PSA) test described in Chapter 5. Because of its ease of use—and despite the uncertainty in its accuracy—PSA testing became widely available starting in the mid-1980s and accepted as a standard screening test with more and more medical professional associations, most notably the American Urological Association, advocating for its use.

But while it is true that prostate cancer cells exude PSA into the bloodstream, where it can be easily found and quantitated, it turns out that *normal* prostate cells also produce *some* PSA. Further, some noncancerous diseases of the prostate, such as infection or the gradual enlargement of the prostate that occurs with age (benign prostatic hypertrophy), also increase the amount of PSA secreted into the bloodstream. Thus, unlike the mammogram, which has a high degree of specificity (meaning that the abnormal patterns of fibrous breast tissue or tiny calcium deposits seen on mammograms are more or less uniquely associated with cancer cells that may metastasize if not dealt with promptly), the PSA test is far less accurate. Indeed, an elevated PSA test is far more likely to be due to noncancerous causes than prostate cancer.

But it gets even worse. If a male patient has an elevated PSA, most physicians recommend a prostate biopsy—usually performed by passing a large needle into the prostate through the wall of the rectum, which abuts the prostate. The tissue samples (so-called "core" biopsies because they resemble the cylinder of earth that is removed during drilling) are separated into tiny slices and examined under the microscope. If clusters of abnormal-appearing cells are seen, they are scored as to deviation from normal prostate—so called "de-differentiation." In fact, most oncologists think of cancer cells as being "nondifferentiated" clones of cells, or cells that for whatever reason fail to mature and perform their normal function. And, of course, one of the normal functions of mature cells in an organ is to remain in place; cancer cells have a tendency not to remain in place, perhaps because they do not bind to other normal cells, and thus metastasize.

We introduced the prostate biopsy grading system in the previous chapter on screening, and it is useful to expand a bit upon it. Recall that biopsy grading system was invented by a physician named Gleason back in the 1980s and has come to be known as the Gleason score.[3] The pathologist looks for five basic patterns that are assigned numbers 1 through 5. They are illustrated again in Figure 6-3.

Since two core samples are reviewed by the pathologist, the pros-

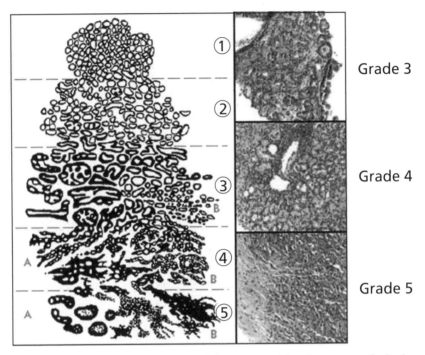

Grade 3

Grade 4

Grade 5

FIGURE 6-3. The pathologist's view of the prostate: How biopsies might look.

tate biopsy score can range from 2 (that is, Grade 1 seen twice) to 10 (that is, Grade 5 seen twice).

It has been well established that the Gleason score *is most certainly* associated with the propensity of an individual's prostate cancer to metastasize, which in turn is by far the major determinant of overall survival.

So you'd think that *if* the tumor was discovered early, *especially* if the Gleason score is high, or *if* the tumor was found at an early "grade" before it progressed into a higher and thus more-likely-to-metastasize grade, the physician would be doing the patient a favor by removing the tumor or killing the tumor cells with large doses of radiation. However, the studies to date involving over 55,000 men with prostate cancer do not validate the hypothesis[4] that early aggressive treatment will save lives. This is very puzzling, no doubt. How is it possible that all this treatment has not lead to better outcomes? Some insight may be obtained if you break down the different types of prostate cancer according to the Gleason scale, and reasons you can start to see that, for many patients, aggressive treatment won't improve the situation. Here are several for which prostate cancer screening with PSA and biopsy may fail to lengthen life:

- For *high-grade* lesions (say, for example, a Gleason score from two core biopsy microscopic examinations of 7 to 10), *some* tumor cells may have already metastasized by the time the tumor is discovered in the gland.

- For *low-grade* lesions (say a Gleason score of 4, which can be made up of one Grade 3 sample and one Grade 1 sample), the tumor may never metastasize at all, meaning that, if the physician urges the patient to have either a radical prostatectomy surgical procedure or high-dose radiation, the patient receives all of the risks (and unpleasant side effects) of these procedures with none of the benefits

- For *intermediate-grade* lesions (4 to 6 on the Gleason scale), the tumor may actually suddenly convert to a much higher-grade lesion by the time a treatment procedure is done and perhaps metastasize. If it does, removing the primary tumor does no good at all; interestingly enough, prostate cancer within the prostate gland itself rarely causes pain, obstruction to urine flow, or any other symptoms of which the patient is aware.

It turns out that, by the time prostate cancer is identified *within* the gland as a result of screening, 15% of the time the tumor has metastasized; we know this only in retrospect, of course, because it is impossible in any individual to see tiny collections of prostate cancer cells in bone, the lungs, or the brain—the primary metastatic sites of this particular cancer—even with our most advanced imaging techniques. The unfortunate story of a man who is two year's postradical prostatectomy having sudden onset of back pain or a collapse of his femur while walking—both due to metastasis of prostate cancer to bones—is a common one in medical offices today. So these are men who endured all the treatment and bad side effects, but their cancers spread anyway.

Put into numerical terms, because about 250,000 cases of prostate cancer are diagnosed by screening every year, about 35,000 of those will have already become metastatic by the time the presumably "early" diagnosis is made. Unfortunately, there is little we can do for these patients except to control pain and treat individual metastases as they occur, typically with radiation therapy to the bone or brain. Longevity over the past 20 years in patients with advanced prostate cancer—defined for our purposes as metastasis of the tumor beyond the prostate gland—hasn't changed much at all.

Of the rest—roughly 200,000—there is precious little evidence that removing the prostate gland made any difference since the prostate cancer would not have metastasized. We await 2011 or 2012 for the results of new studies in progress for the past eight years or so to tell us who benefits most from prostate cancer screening. These studies may also tell us who should *not* have prostate cancer screening, because for some groups of men the PSA test may be particularly problematic in falsely identifying those who require biopsy and treatment.

WHAT ABOUT OTHER CANCERS'
INCIDENCE RATES AND PROGNOSES?

We have seen that screening for prostate cancer—unlike that for breast cancer in females—has made no demonstrable difference in longevity or survival. What about other cancers in males and females? A recent review[3] puts into clear, quantitative terms the successes and failures we have had.

First, to the extent that there has been a decrease in the overall death rate per year from cancer, almost all of that improvement is explained by two factors: (1) widespread use of mammography for detecting and treating early forms of breast cancer; (2) a reduction in the use of cigarettes. The latter is clearly responsible for most of the decrease in male lung cancer and for some cases of bladder cancer (much rarer). Unfortunately, we cannot say how many of the "early" breast cancers identified in women might have never metastasized (or, indeed, might have spontaneously disappeared). But, unlike prostate cancer screening in males, it is at least clear that women's lives have been saved, and usually with fewer side effects as our surgical techniques have become much more targeted—removing the breast cancer lump rather than the entire breast—and that our chemotherapy is much less toxic in the case of breast cancer. (Of course, that is not to say that having breast cancer is a walk in the park—it certainly is not easy for any woman with the disease!)

Second, some behaviors known to increase the risk of cancer have, regrettably, *increased*. The clearest example is the increased rate of smoking in young women in spite of admonitions from various surgeons-general of the United States and physicians about the dangers of smoking. Thus, lung cancer rates (and deaths from lung cancer, one of the many cancers that is generally incurable) have increased among females.

Third, while it *appears* that survival times in patients diagnosed with cancers have increased, it is *not* clear whether this is merely a result of diagnosing the tumor earlier *or* of our therapies being more effective against early stages of metastatic tumor than more advanced stages. While it is tempting to conclude that chemotherapeutic and radiation therapies would be expected to work better if the total cancer burden is smaller (that is, the tumor is at an earlier stage), this remains to be demonstrated even after millions of cases and thousands of papers analyzing the data from those cases have been published. It is most likely that we are simply diagnosing cancer earlier, thus "starting the clock" at an earlier time before death supervenes, giving the false impression that we are increasing survival times in patients with cancer.

Finally, more than half of all cancers are now diagnosed in people over the age of 65, a percentage that is much higher than even 20 years ago. Because of the aging population, this trend is likely to continue. Thus, we will probably see more cancer diagnoses—albeit in older people—simply because people are living longer. The latter, of course, is not necessarily a bad thing as long as the extra years people are living do not result in painful and/or unpleasant treatment for cancer, which at one time was rare in people over 65, just because there weren't many people over that age.

Clearly, the primary goal in cancer control is to prevent cancer from occurring in the first place, primarily by reducing smoking rates in the population. But if we fail at prevention, advances in early detection and treatment may someday change cancer into a manageable chronic—but not fatal—disease. But we haven't gotten there yet.

SOME HOPEFUL NEWS FROM THE FRONT ON THE WAR ON CANCER: WHAT MIGHT BE AROUND THE CORNER

It is helpful to review our progress pictorially as a window on recent advances in our understanding of the biology of cells—cancer cells included—that could make a meaningful difference in minimizing the harm from unnecessary screening and perhaps improving specific therapy for cancer on an individual basis.

The National Cancer Institute has calculated the number of lives saved in the year 2000, compared with 1990, from just about all of the known types of cancer. Their results are presented in Figure 6-4. Let's look at the five cancers that account for 90% of all cancers: (1) lung cancer (in both males and females), (2) breast cancer in females, (3) prostate cancer in males, and (4) colon and (5) stomach cancer (for both males and females).

It is important to understand that the dramatic number of "lives saved" from lung cancer in males comes not as a result of advances in the treatment of lung cancer but rather in the *prevention* of lung cancer. The latter is due almost exclusively to the reduction in smoking among males and is further proven by what is happening in the female population: an *increase* in lung cancer deaths—or as Figure 6-4 puts it, a "negative" number of lives saved—because women are smoking more now than they did 20 or 25 years ago. It is terribly frustrating to public health officials and physicians that modern advertising has made smoking seem both attractive and safe among young females. After all, those ads for Virginia Slims cigarettes always show very well dressed, pretty females with smiles on their faces as a cancer-inducing stick dangles subtly from their fingers.

The estimates for (male) lives saved from prostate cancer is based on the *assumption* that a substantial percentage of the prostate cancers

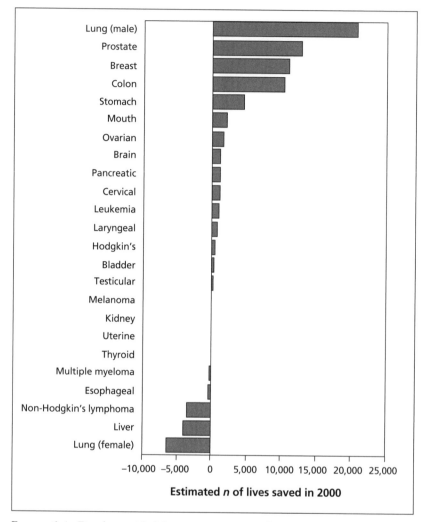

FIGURE 6-4. Deaths avoided from various types of cancers in 2000, compared to 1990. (Source: National Cancer Institute.)

discovered by screening *would in fact have become metastatic disease.* But, as noted earlier, this is a highly questionable assumption.

Mammographic screening for breast cancer is our single biggest success (save for decreased smoking in males) in preventing deaths from cancer. Colon *polyp* screening has helped reduce the precursors to colon cancer, and it is likely that, as screening becomes more widely accepted, more colon cancer deaths will be avoided. The costs, however, are enormous since a colonoscopy exam costs on the order of $2,500 (not including lost days of work for the patients). And, as a lesson in the unexpected (which is the rule in modern medicine), stomach cancer deaths are decreasing, due neither to screening nor to better treatment but rather to better treatment of stomach ulcers, which are believed to be the precursors to most stomach cancers (but it is essential to note that the overwhelming majority of stomach ulcers never lead to cancer). Thus, better drugs for the treatment of a painful but usually benign condition—stomach ulcers—had the unexpected side effect of reducing the incidence of stomach cancer. It is also likely that dietary changes, with many people avoiding heavily smoked or preserved meats and moving to fish and a higher vegetable diet, have reduced stomach cancer incidence as well.

All of these benefits taken into consideration, it is possible to quantify the increase in longevity and quality of life due to treatment per se in the four or five major cancers of adults that have become metastatic. For metastatic breast cancer, there is general agreement that quality of life is better now than 20 years ago, and longevity has increased by about a year. Similar results have been seen in some of the subtypes of lung cancer and colon cancer, but probably not with prostate or stomach cancer, let alone rarer cancers. In short, in those patients with metastatic disease from common cancers, increases in longevity have amounted to a few months to a year or so. An advance to be sure, but modest.

Finally, for the rare cancers—those dozens of cancer types that together make up less than 10% of all cancer diagnoses—there is little new to say. Once they are metastatic, ovarian, brain, pancreatic, esophageal, and cervical cancers completely defy medical therapy. Survival from metastatic colon, lung, breast, ovarian, and skin cancers of various types are about the same now as they were in the 1970s: about 25,000 deaths per year for each type.

With rare exception, the only significant progress we've made in the "war" is in the prevention of cancer from screening and from decreases in cigarette consumption (at least in males). None of this is to say that meaningful advances in the treatment of the most common cancers that have escaped early detection and become metastatic will not be realized, but it is key for patients to understand that our approaches to date—based mostly on chemotherapy that kills more cancer cells but also carries with it more side effects—have yielded much marginal benefit. It is essential for the individual to discuss with their physician the trade-offs of increased toxicity and modest (if any) increase in survival.

Although it will take time to realize, there is clearly new hope in the treatment of cancer—and even the decisions to *not* treat some cancers such as localized prostate cancer in males—based on an ever more thorough understanding of the genetic changes in specific cancer types. Because it is now possible to sequence and characterize the entirety of the genome in cancer cells from specific patients (which used to take weeks, and now can be accomplished in hours), data from thousands of cancer patients is being accumulated that will answer fundamental questions that have been unanswered for decades: Is the most common type of breast (or prostate, lung, or colon) cancer as seen under the microscope more than just one disease? And if so, what is its behavior likely to be in a given individual? Can the immune system be used in a very selective way to attack and eliminate cancer cells of certain types?

Preliminary data already suggests that we can already be more selective in the intensity of chemotherapy for certain sub-sets of breast cancer patients with metastatic disease, sparing toxicity and increasing the efficacy of treatment regimens, and similar results are expected for the other common cancer types in adults. Thus, manipulating the genes of cancer cells is now a reality, albeit on small scale, and it represents a dramatic shift in the way metastatic cancer will be managed and perhaps cured in the majority of cases. And there *may* lie the answers we have sought for the past four decades.

NOTES

1. A fascinating video and audio history of this event is available on the Web site of the National Institutes of Health at http://dtp.nci.nih.gov/timeline/noflash/

milestones/M4_Nixon.htm. The U.S Army's biological warfare facility at Ft. Detrick, Maryland was largely devoted to carrying out the National Cancer Act of 1971, with laboratories once dedicated to developing weapons based on biological organisms converted to finding the cure for cancer. Little did anyone know at the time how difficult the job would be or even that cancer is not one disease but a multitude of different diseases that depend inherently on a few changes in the DNA that directs the function of specific cell types.

2. Everyone is familiar with the amazing story of Greg LeMonde, seven-time winner of the Tour de France bicycle race who had testicular cancer that had spread widely throughout his body—to his lungs and brain. Intensive radiation and chemotherapy not only cured him, it was handled so well (and LeMonde was otherwise in such good shape to survive it all) that he triumphed again in what has to be one of the most demanding and grueling of all endurance races. LeMonde appears regularly on television commercials (for the company that makes some of the chemotherapeutic drugs his doctors used), touting the dramatic advances in cancer treatment. But since testicular cancer is rare, Lemond's experience is also rare.

3. D. F. Gleason, "Histologic grade, clinical stage, and patient age in prostate cancer," *National Cancer Institute Monograph 7*, 1988: 15–18.

4. F. Labrie, B. Candas, L. Cusan, J. L. Gomez, A. Belanger, G. Brousseau, E. Chevrette, and J. Leveseque, "Screening decreases prostate cancer mortality: 11-year follow-up of the 1988 Quebec prospective randomized controlled trial." *Prostate*, 2004; 59(3): 311–318; 2000; 284(18): 2313–2314; and G. Sandblom, E, Varenhorst, O. Lofman, J. Rosell, and P. Carlsson, "Clinical consequences of screening for prostate cancer: 15 years follow-up of a randomised controlled trial in Sweden." *European Urology*, 2004; 46: 717–724.

5. Patrick L. Remington and Amy Trentham-Dietz, "Measuring progress in cancer control: A bird's eye view," *The Oncologist*, December 2003; 8(6): 539–540.

CHAPTER 7

Diabetes: Things You May Not Know

THE CENTERS FOR DISEASE CONTROL estimates that about 8% (one person out of 12) of the adult population in the United States has diabetes, and almost a third don't know that they do. Large textbooks and at least a dozen major medical journals are devoted to the study and understanding of diabetes, so only a bit of the science of diabetes will be covered in this chapter. Instead, we'll focus on the complications of diabetes that cause symptoms and organ dysfunction, along with the treatments available. Unsurprisingly, there is very little evidence that, despite 50 years of treating the disease, any of the treatments do much good. Some, indeed, probably do a great deal of harm.

WHAT IS DIABETES?

Diabetes is a "metabolic" disorder, specifically a disease associated with the uptake and disposition of nutrients in one's diet. By definition, diabetes is diagnosed when one of three abnormalities in the blood level of glucose is detected:

1. First, in individuals who have the classical symptoms of diabetes such as excessive thirst, increased urination, and sudden weight loss, if the blood sugar is greater than 200 milligrams per 10 cubic centimeters of plasma (normal is between 55 and 100 milligrams per 10 cubic centimeters of plasma).[1] This turns out to be the *least* common way physicians identify patients with diabetes.
2. Second, in any individual whose "fasting" blood sugar is greater than 126 milligrams per deciliter (mg/dl). "Fasting" is defined as having no caloric intake of any kind for eight hours or more.
3. Third, in individuals who drink a sugary slurry of glucose (75 grams of glucose dissolved in water) and who have a blood sugar of greater than 200 mg/dl two hours later. This test is called the "oral glucose tolerance test" (OGTT) and isn't used routinely except in evaluating women who became diabetic during pregnancy to see if they have a tendency to become chronically diabetic.

Glucose is one of the body's primary fuels. The brain and most blood cells are completely dependent on it, and other organs, such as the muscles and the liver, function optimally with it. Interestingly, the primary fuel that the heart uses is fat; the heart depends almost not at all on having a supply of glucose to function efficiently.

The primary dietary source of glucose is carbohydrates—what most of us call either "starchy" foods (like bread and pasta) and "sugary-tasting" foods (like soft drinks, and candy). In reality, just about any food we eat has some carbohydrate content save for pure fats (like cooking oils or shortening). Meat contains carbohydrates, but also contains protein.

Since many of the organs of the body depend on glucose almost exclusively for normal function, even in the absence of any intake of carbohydrates, the liver can make glucose out of other nutrients, primarily proteins from some vegetables, meats, fish, and egg albumin. Thus, even if one consumes zero carbohydrates (which is just about impossible), glucose is always available as long as protein is being eaten.

But the real key to understanding of diabetes isn't the blood sugar measurement per se, even though that's how the diagnosis is made in the physician's office, but rather the effects of glucose that is, on average, above normal. Even in people without diabetes, the glucose level varies quite a bit throughout the day, though by definition it seldom if ever gets above about 125 to 130 mg/dl. In patients with diabetes, whose blood sugar is frequently above 130 mg/dl and may be for long periods of time, glucose appears to do damage to cells throughout the body. The mechanisms are complex and incompletely understood, but when cells are bathed in excess glucose, their own internal metabolism changes, and the cells—and thus the organs that are made up of billions of cells—are often damaged.

We'll look at the details of the chronic effects of diabetes, but first a bit more information on how glucose is normally used and what we believe makes that process go awry.

THE USE AND ABUSE OF GLUCOSE

When you sit down to a plate of your favorite pasta, an amazing series of events takes place, starting right away in your mouth, that converts that dried-wheat-from-the-fields-of-Italy into the most important fuel that cells all over your body need. Wheat kernels are carbohydrates, which, when made into pasta are long chemical chains of glucose and closely related molecules all linked together. These huge chains may be made of hundreds of millions of glucose molecules, far too large to be absorbed by the tiny cells in the gastrointestinal tract. It is helpful to follow the course of a delicious meal from plate to fate to get some insights into glucose metabolism and diabetes.

Enzymes are specialized molecules secreted by cells that catalyze (speed up) or carry out very specific reactions. In the digestion of pasta (or related foods), several dozen have been identified that help break down the big carbohydrate molecules into usable fuel. The first major enzyme, called amylase, is poured into your mouth by your salivary glands. Amylase begins breaking the chemical bonds in the chain of glucose (and closely similar) chemicals that make up your meal.

In the stomach, the acidic environment works mostly on digesting proteins and doesn't help much with the further breakdown of carbohydrates. So, as the now partially digested pasta passes into the small intestine, it still can't be absorbed by the billions of cells in the intestine because the molecules of the once-pasta are still too large. Enter the pancreas, which secretes even more amylase into the intestines, along with a half-dozen other enzymes secreted by the cells lining the intestines. The once huge molecules that made up pasta are now reduced to one-, two-, or three-glucose molecules strung together. These "simple" sugars are sometimes called "mono-," "di-," or "tri-saccharides" (for one-, two-, or three-glucose—or very similar—molecules linked together). These are small enough to be absorbed.

Once in the bloodstream, the simple sugars are immediately taken up by some cells of the brain, kidney, and white cells to use as fuel. Actively exercising muscle can also use them, and indeed glucose and its close cousins are most easily converted into actual "work" or movement by muscles. When sprinters are at their top speed, their leg muscles are using mostly glucose.

Interestingly, for all intents and purposes, all of the cell types just mentioned can absorb glucose passively (by diffusion) from the blood. But other organs require a critical hormone called *insulin*—made exclusively in specialized cells of the pancreas, which are distinct from the ones that make digestive enzymes—in order to use glucose. The most important organ in this regard is the liver, which, in the presence of circulating insulin and glucose, absorbs the latter and reassembles it into a special carbohydrate called glycogen, essentially another huge chain of glucose molecules, effectively reversing the digestion and breakdown of ingested carbohydrates. Conversely, in the middle of the night when it has been hours since you've eaten anything, the liver breaks down the glycogen with its own specialized enzyme system and releases glucose molecules back into the bloodstream because they are the "soul food" for the brain and blood cells.

So your pasta meal or carbohydrate-laden dessert is broken down into countless tiny glucose molecules, absorbed by the upper part of the small intestine, and then distributed via the bloodstream to organs that absolutely require glucose. Anything not immediately used by these organs is absorbed by the liver (and also by nonexercising muscle) *if* insulin is present. And that's where the trouble begins, leading to the disease known as diabetes.

TWO TYPES OF DIABETES

Diabetes is really two (and perhaps more) separate diseases. If insulin production stops entirely—and when this happens, the reasons for it are usually unclear—the liver and resting muscles, which are the storage areas for almost all of the glucose in the body, can't absorb glucose from the bloodstream. The blood sugar obviously rises. At the same time, however, the liver cells and muscles have to have *something* to live on; they can't go without fuel. And when the preferred fuel, glucose, can't get into cells, muscles, and liver, the body's cells start using fat.

That would be a good thing in general (since everyone wants to lose fat) except that, when there is no insulin at all around, the process of breaking down fat for use as a fuel occurs suddenly and in huge quantities. And, for reasons that are complex, every time fat is broken down, some amount of acid is released into the bloodstream. If that happens quickly enough, the blood becomes saturated with fat and acid—a condition known as "ketoacidosis" (with "keto" being short for "ketone," a breakdown product of fat stores).

It is important to understand that, with very rare exception, ketoacidosis occurs only in the total (or nearly total) absence of insulin. As one might imagine, highly acidic blood interferes with the function of cells all over the body that are designed to operate in a very tightly regulated environment of limited amounts of free-floating acid. Thus, in ketoacidosis patients, the symptoms are not subtle: multiple organs begin to fail, the patient may lose consciousness because the neurons in the brain are exquisitely sensitive to changes in blood acid content, and death may supervene in minutes to hours.

Before insulin was isolated, studied, and then first used as a therapeutic agent back in the 1920s, just about every person with ketoacidosis—or, more correctly diabetic ketoacidosis (DKA)—died. When the first person with DKA was treated with insulin and saved, a major medical miracle was realized (and the Nobel Prize was bestowed on the Canadians Frederick Banting and Charles Best, along with Scottish physiologist John Macleod, for isolating and purifying it). Even today, DKA is treated first and foremost with insulin.

Type I diabetes—a relatively rare disorder—refers to elevated blood sugar levels (and almost always DKA as well sometime in its course) that occur due to the *absence* of any insulin production. It is a disease most commonly seen in young people, the vast majority between the ages of 5 and 16. We know that the specialized cells in the pancreas that produce insulin stop functioning; we don't know why, but the speculation among most researchers is that the body's own immune system destroys those cells. Why the latter happens remains a mystery.

Patients with Type I diabetes on rare occasion recover function of the pancreas cells—called "beta cells"—that make insulin. But more than 98% are forever dependent on insulin to keep immediately life-threatening DKA at bay and to keep the blood sugar levels within reasonable ranges. Extreme fluctuations or chronically elevated blood sugar levels do chronic damage, as we'll see.

Fortunately, Type I diabetes is uncommon. The vast majority of diabetics—called Type II diabetics—don't suffer from an absolute lack of insulin but rather appear to develop a relative *resistance* to insulin. While their pancreases pour out insulin in quantities usually *above* normal, the liver, muscle, and other cells dependent upon it to absorb glucose don't respond optimally. Once again, the mechanisms are complex and very poorly understood. But, distinct from Type I diabetics, the much-more common Type II diabetics generally have no lack of insulin, but their bodies' cells just don't use the insulin very well.

Type II diabetes is almost always diagnosed in adults over the age of 45 who are almost always overweight or frankly obese (more than 30% over ideal body weight). These patients tend to be physically inactive (though by no means is this always the case), and they also have other significant medical problems, which physicians call "co-moridities," most often high blood pressure and markedly elevated cholesterol levels. Because so many things are wrong in Type II diabetes patients, physicians often say they have a "metabolic syndrome," meaning that many aspects of normal body and cell functions have gone awry.

In all diabetics the most important parameter to follow is, of course, the blood sugar. Symptoms that patients report are doubtless also taken into account by most good doctors when they are treating patients, but there can be little doubt that it is glucose level that matters supremely to the doctor—and sometimes even to insurance companies that review physician performance in treating diabetes.

As already hinted at earlier, both wild swings in glucose and in the average level of glucose reflect the degree of control of the diabetes. Measuring the blood glucose at any given moment is easy but may not represent what is happening most of the time, unless the physician obtains multiple blood samples over many days—something most patients don't like to do or won't. Thus, a major breakthrough about 20 years ago occurred when a test became available that could be given by doctors and patients and that gave a good idea of how much of the time the glucose was elevated too much. The test, called the A1C hemoglobin, takes advantage of a physiologic fact: when the oxygen-carrying molecule called hemoglobin (found almost exclusively inside red blood cells) is bathed in glucose, some of that glucose irreversibly binds to the hemoglobin. When hemoglobin is combined with glucose, the hemoglobin is termed "glycosylated"—abbreviated as HA1C.[3] In nondiabetic people, about 6% of the all hemoglobin has glucose bound to it; in diabetics, that number can easily exceed 10%. The important point is that, once glucose binds to hemoglobin, it stays there until the red blood cell carrying the hemoglobin reaches the end of its life span—about four to five months. So, to put this information into perspective, the HA1C reflects the average level of glucose over about four months—quite different from a random glucose measurement that may be normal or wildly abnormal in a diabetic.

When the HA1C was available for physicians to use as a test, several long-term trials of treatment of diabetes were begun, using this reading as the single best measurement available for the long-term control of diabetes. And we now know that HA1C levels are well correlated with the incidence of coronary artery disease in patients with diabetes and less certainly with the incidence of other complications.

But, as we shall see, that doesn't mean that *lowering* the HA1C with medications results in a lowering of complications. As is frequently the case in medicine, just because one can measure a laboratory abnormality, reversing that abnormality doesn't necessarily result in better health or treatment outcomes.

GLUCOSE: THE SMALL MOLECULE THAT'S A BIG DEAL

So, putting aside the relatively rare Type I diabetics who will die without regular insulin injections,[4] why all the fuss about elevated blood sugars in the 21 million American adults with Type II diabetes? The answer is that chronic elevations of glucose do much damage to tiny blood vessels (the microvascular effects of diabetes) and to large blood vessels (macrovascular effects). The results in terms of suffering or symptoms are very different, and for reasons that remain completely obscure, some Type II diabetes patients get both kinds of adverse effects and others get one or the other.

Microvascular disease manifests itself primarily in three organs: the eyes, the kidneys, and probably the heart. In the eyes (which technically speaking are part of the brain, so doctors are quick to point out that small blood vessels in the brain can be similarly affected), the many millions of tiny blood vessels in the retina of the eye start to leak. Proteins, fluids, and other constituents from the blood cause the retina to swell. (See Figure 7-1.) Then, since the retina itself is made up of the light-sensitive cells that are the basis of vision, diabetics frequently have many visual symptoms: loss of acuity, loss of color

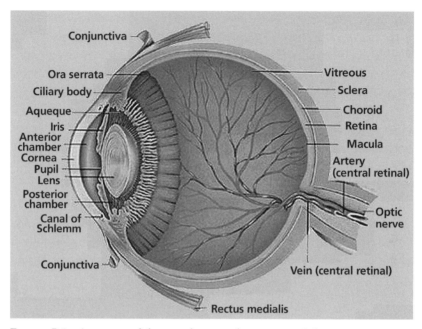

Conjunctiva

Ora serrata
Ciliary body
Aqueque
Iris
Anterior chamber
Cornea
Pupil
Lens
Posterior chamber
Canal of Schlemm

Conjunctiva

Rectus medialis

Vitreous
Sclera
Choroid
Retina
Macula
Artery (central retinal)

Optic nerve

Vein (central retinal)

FIGURE 7-1. Anatomy of the eye showing the retina and the vitreous.

vision, and sometimes complete blindness. The latter can occur when the tiny blood vessels leak so badly that blood pours out in such a large quantity that it can cause damage in several ways. It can cover large portions of the retina, causing the jelly-like material that makes up most of the eye (the vitreous humor[5]) to detach from the retina, destroying irreplaceable retinal cells in the process. Or, perhaps surprisingly, when the body attempts to clean up the red blood cells and sends in white blood cells to mop up the mess, delicate retinal cells are irreversibly damaged in the process. This specific manifestation of small vessel disease in the eye in diabetics is called "diabetic retinopathy." Its severity varies tremendously from one individual to another, and usually it takes about a decade after on the onset of Type II diabetes for the retina to begin to suffer.

In the kidney, a similar process takes place in the million or so extremely delicate filters called "glomeruli." These are made up of microscopic blood vessels that are selectively porous in normal function: waste matter passes through the vessels and is collected into the urine, but useful constituents of the blood—proteins, antibodies, clotting factors, and myriad other molecules—are retained to be returned to the bloodstream. In *diabetic nephropathy*, much like diabetic retinopathy, the glomerular blood vessels leak normal constituents into the urine. In addition, the cells that make up the glomeruli start to die—once again, the precise mechanism is unknown—become sclerotic, and disappear from the kidney. Carried to its logical conclusion over several million glomeruli, the kidneys fail to do their job. Diabetes is by far the most common cause of renal failure in the United States.

In large blood vessels such as the aorta, the coronary arteries, or the arteries that supply blood to the legs and brain, a different process takes place as a result (at least in part) to the elevated blood sugar found in Type II diabetics: acceleration of atherosclerosis. While just about everybody who lives long enough develops some degree of narrowing of large arteries due to cholesterol deposits and the subsequent, unsuccessful attempt of the body to repair or remove the deposits, diabetics have this problem almost uniformly and with much greater severity than similarly aged people without diabetes. As a result, heart attacks and stroke are much, much more common in diabetics than in nondiabetics who are otherwise of the same age, race, weight, and gender.

SHOULD HIGH GLUCOSE LEVELS BE FIXED?

From all of the detailed discussion of physiology and glucose metabolism, it would be logical to conclude that, if elevated blood glucose levels could be controlled—preferably so that they were normal all of the time—both microvascular and macrovascular complications would disappear or be much reduced. So, for years, physicians (and especially those doctors who work in the subspecialty field of endocrinology) have been trying various interventions to bring blood sugar levels down in patients with Type II diabetes. It turns out that, while there are many ways to lower blood sugar, few have been shown to make any difference in preventing the micro- or macrovascular problems so common in diabetics. Let's review those interventions.

First, exercise and weight loss (either together or separately) clearly result in lower blood sugar levels on average and also "peak" blood sugar measurements after eating. More important, this simple intervention has been unequivocally shown to decrease the probability of both small and large vessel disease in newly diagnosed diabetics. If one follows, over 10 or 20 years, a typical, overweight, 50-year-old American with elevated blood sugars who loses the excess weight via dieting or exercise (and preferably both), the likelihood of eye, kidney or heart disease or of gangrene of the extremities due to advanced atherosclerosis of the large blood vessels is reduced to roughly the same risk as that of the nondiabetic patient. And with the weight loss comes normalization of blood sugars.

Based on this experience, it would be tempting to conclude that, for patients who won't or can't lose weight or exercise, if physicians could lower the blood sugar with medications, the incidence of coronary disease or other vascular complications of diabetes would be reduced. But, by and large, that logic doesn't work out in real life. For example, one can give Type II diabetics extra insulin to take, which, in most people, brings down peak blood sugar levels. And, if insulin is taken before every meal, the average blood sugar can be brought down to normal. Unfortunately—and for reasons we don't understand—despite improving the overall level of blood sugar control, long-term studies show that, if one does so using insulin, the incidence of vascular disease is actually *worse* than if no insulin is used at all.

So, if insulin isn't the answer in Type II diabetics, what about oral medications? In the 1940s through the 1960s, several drugs were serendipitously discovered that lowered blood sugar. They were originally intended for much different purposes, such as treating infection, and were found to have this unexpected side effect. There are several classes of these drugs, generally referred to as "oral hypoglycemic agents," which we will briefly review. Note that they are not in any way related to insulin or derived from it. They should not be thought of as "oral insulin" medications, a misnomer sometimes blurted out by physicians and other health care providers.

Sulfonylureas

First is the *sulfonylureas*. These drugs, derivatives of the sulfa drugs of the World War II era and among the first antibiotics, were found to cause hypoglycemia (low blood sugar) in experimental animals. As so often happens in medicine, this was a purely chance discovery. One of the sulfonylureas—tolbutamide—was introduced in the 1950s as a medication for Type II diabetes and is still in use today along with about two dozen other similar compounds. Doubtless some people reading this chapter are taking tolbutamide or one of its cousins.

Sulfonylureas work, at least partially, by causing the pancreatic beta cells to produce more insulin. There is no question that they lower blood sugar, but they seem to do so at a price: increased weight (after all, that glucose ends up somewhere and can even be converted into fat if too much is stored) and eventual loss of potency. There is some evidence that microvascular complications can be delayed but not entirely prevented by use of these drugs.

Biguanides

The second class of oral diabetes are the *biguanides*. They are named from the guanidine, a constituent of DNA that was accidentally found, to cause blood sugar to fall when it was given in large doses intravenously to mice. Incredible as it may sound, this discovery was made in 1918—even before DNA was known. Guanidine itself works poorly as an oral hypoglycemic agent in humans, but two derivatives of guanidine found their way into the marketplace, one of which—metformin (also called by its trade name, Glucophage)—is widely in use today.

Metformin works differently than the sulfonylureas; it does not lead to an increase in the release of insulin but rather seems to sensitize cells to the effects of insulin already being produced by the pancreas. In other words, metformin overcomes what appears to be the fundamental problem in Type II diabetes: insulin resistance at the cellular level. More than any other oral drug we have today, metformin has the best track record for reducing both macrovascular and microvascular disease, but again, as time goes on, it loses its potency in keeping blood sugars down.

Thiazolidinediones (TZDs)

The third, and most recent class of oral hypoglycemics, goes by the tongue-twisting name of *thiazolidinediones* (*TZDs*). Most patients know them by their trade names: Avandia, Actos, and a few others. These drugs—introduced in the 1990s but again discovered more or less by accident—were thought to avoid the weight gain of sulfonylureas and the loss of potency with time that the other two classes of oral hypogly-cemic drugs suffered from. And, when first introduced, TZDs appeared to meet those promises and more: they were thought to be especially good at being cardioprotective by reducing vascular disease, especially macrovascular disease. Of course, as new agents on pharmacy shelves, they are very expensive: as much as 50 times as expensive as the older sulfonylureas or metformin.

But as with most things that seem to be too good to be true, the TZDs have turned out to be a disaster. After a few years of use, it became clear that the TZDs have a nasty tendency to cause heart failure via a mechanism that appears to be due to its effects on the coronary arteries and on the cells that make up the heart muscle itself.[6] One TZD has actually been withdrawn from the market. Most TZDs eventually cause weight gain.

The Effects of Treatment

At present, it appears that few of the carefully controlled, large clinical trials of the treatment of diabetes have shown much benefit. We be-lieve that this is in large part because the effort to control glucose levels simply wasn't intensive enough. It is, indeed, *possible* to control glucose levels very closely with frequent measurements of blood sugar, multiple doses of insulin, and ever increasing doses of metformin or other oral hypoglycemic agents. But not only has there been no benefit yet shown of intensive treatment in Type II diabetics (aside from the clear benefits of weight loss and exercise), there are several costs in lives and dollars:

- The more intensively one treats diabetes with medications, the greater the risk is for *too low* of a blood sugar (hypoglyce-mia), which can result in death.

- The costs of home glucose testing three to five times a day is several hundred dollars a month (plus the pain of lots of nee-dle poking of the fingers).

- The costs of medications plus treatment for hypoglycemia are enormous—many billions of extra dollars a year.

Finally, most physicians will tell you that, despite all of the admonition, counseling, and education they can muster—which also costs lots of money for additional physician and diabetic educator fees—they just can't get most patients to do what the ADA suggests.

Recommendations for "tight" or "intensive" control of diabetes gets a grade of E, meaning "no controlled studies suggest this works, but experts believe it might." As we've seen so many times in the recent history of medicine, experts, as well intentioned as they may be, are often wrong. If we've learned anything at all about diabetes in the past 50 years it is this: it is simply naïve to think that diabetes is all or even mostly about an elevated blood sugar that needs to be beaten down to normal. The disorder is much more complex than that because we know that, for most diabetics, the lion's share of the benefits of treatment of blood sugar per se—and they are modest—come from lowering the extremes of blood sugar, not from lowering the HA1C from 8% to 6%. The latter goal is not only unattainable in the real world; attaining it doesn't help much, and it puts patients at risk for life-threatening complications.

Thus, the lessons learned from new therapies in cardiology, for the treatment of various cancers and other common maladies apply to diabetes as well: simple logic doesn't apply well in biology, probably because the mechanisms of disease are far more complex than even the most advanced diagnostic and experimental tests can tell us. The *only* approach that makes sense is a careful, controlled therapeutic trial done for a sufficient period of time—usually years—so that unexpected adverse side effects can be revealed.

For diabetes, we've learned that the control of blood sugar is important and meaningful in terms of preventing complications *if* the blood sugar is lowered by diet with weight loss or exercise (and preferably both). Similar reductions in blood sugar by medications aren't nearly as successful in preventing the complications of diabetes (which, in the end, is what cause both terrible disease and suffering during life and which also lead to early death). To the extent that medications do work, the old inexpensive ones (Metformin at about $5 per month) are both safer and at least as efficacious as the new (but obviously inadequately tested) drugs that have been held out as a marvel of pharmacology but that to date have caused more harm than good.

SO WHAT MAKES SENSE FOR PATIENTS WITH TYPE II DIABETES?

Many millions of people in the United States have diabetes, and many more are projected to have it as poorer societies around the world become wealthier and gain access to Western-type diets rich in calories, let alone cholesterol.[7] It is therefore obviously important to identify the interventions that prolong the quality and quantity of life for diabetics while we await a clear set of proven treatments for diabetes.

First and foremost are exercise and weight loss. There is no risk to this approach, it has demonstrated efficacy in preventing complications, and the cost is low. Unfortunately, most people won't adhere to a regular exercise regime.

Next is a *reasonable* control of blood sugar. If random blood sugar readings are three times normal or if the HA1C is four or five percentage points above the normal of 5% or 6%, then lowering those numbers with medication gives some modest benefit in terms of preventing some of the complications of diabetes. Pushing any harder does little, if any, good and has a high probability of causing harm.

But there is some good news, though it has nothing to do with blood sugar per se. Most Type II diabetics have abnormalities in cholesterol and blood pressure, and it is abundantly clear from many well controlled studies that controlling these two measurements *does* result in increased longevity and reduction in strokes and heart attacks, including in diabetic patients. So the most important thing that adults with diabetes can do to keep their blood pressure and cholesterol in the normal range. The benefits from this usually inexpensive and almost uniformly effective drug regimen *have*—unlike intensive treatment of blood glucose levels—made a positive difference.

Finally, if the intensive control of blood pressure and cholesterol, in addition to reasonable control of blood sugar, is to work, a substantial amount of effort must be put into patient education.[8] Currently the standard of such education is a team of dieticians and nurses who do the lion's share of the follow-up, encouragement, and answering questions. This adds substantially to the cost of treatment, and to date, the cost-effectiveness of the intensive approach remains unknown.[9] Patient preferences—particularly in older patients who may not wish to be bothered with taking yet more pills or injecting more insulin—dramatically influence the cost-effectiveness of almost any approach to the treatment of Type II diabetes, which can easily become, for many people,[10] unwieldy and costly. Both individuals and health care policy planners should bear in mind that the *prevention* of diabetes through lifestyle intervention—primarily done by counseling—is unquestionably cost-effective by the usual metrics of "dollars spent and effort expended per year of high quality life gained."[11]

For diabetic patients who depend on their physicians to help them do the right things, the bottom lines are clear: first, ask to have your cholesterol levels and blood pressure monitored and treated. Second, if you can't or won't lose weight and exercise, ask your doctor to follow carefully the ongoing trials of new medications in the treatment of diabetes, but not to worry—or make you worry—if your blood sugar is a bit out of whack. You can't make it perfect, and even if you do, it almost certainly will do more harm than good.

NOTES

1. Plasma is the portion of blood that does not contain red blood cells and that is easily separated from the blood cells by spinning a sample of whole blood in a centrifuge.
2. "Milligrams per 100 cc of plasma" is usually abbreviated as mg/dl, where "dl" means deciliter or one-tenth of a liter, the same as 100 cubic centimeters (cc) of plasma.
3. Technically, this is written in the literature as HA_{1C}, with the "C" referring the third variant in chemical structure of the dominant type of hemoglobin in red blood cells.
4. Insulin is a very large protein molecule that, as a drug, cannot be taken orally because stomach acid breaks it down or otherwise inactivates it. Thus, insulin

must be given by injection although there is one—and long awaited—inhalable form of insulin that is absorbed in the lungs where acid and enzymes don't destroy it. Unfortunately, the latter has proven problematic and as of this writing is being taken off of the market even though more than two decades of research and billions of dollars went into its development and production.

5. "Humor" in the medical context is derived from the Latin word umorem, which means moisture.

6. "Long-term risk of cardiovascular events with rosiglitazone: a meta-analysis," *Journal of the American Medical Association*, September 2007:12;298(10):1189–95.

7. Diabetes was, until recently virtually unheard of in sub-Saharan Africa and in most of the Far East. Most experts believe that the prevalence of diabetes in the rest of the world will eventually catch up to its level of presence in the United States, though there is nothing new about this observation. We know that very few American Indians had diabetes until the mid-twentieth century when Western habits and diets found their way into Native American populations. Obesity became the rule rather than the exception among adult Native Americans (and now Native American children), and diabetes soon followed. In the Southwestern United States among the Zuni and Navajo Indians, at least one-third of the entire adult population is now diabetic.

8. Peter Gæde, Pernille Vedel, Nicolai Larsen Gunnar V. H. Jensen, Hans-Henrik Parving, and Oluf Pedersen, "Multifactorial intervention and cardiovascular disease in patients with Type 2 diabetes," *New England Journal of Medicine*, 2003; 348: 383–393.

9. K. Dalziel and L. Segal, "Time to give nutrition interventions a higher profile: cost-effectiveness of 10 nutrition interventions," *Health Promotion International*, October 4, 2007.

10. E. S. Huang, M. Shook, L. Jin, M. H. Chin, D. O. Meltzer, "The impact of patient preferences on the cost-effectiveness of intensive glucose control in older patients with new-onset diabetes," *Diabetes Care*, February 2006 ;29(2): 259–264.

11. P. Lindgren, J. Lindström, J. Tuomilehto, M. Uusitupa, M. Peltonen, B. Jönsson, U. de Faire, M. L. Hellénius , DPS Study Group, "Lifestyle intervention to prevent diabetes in men and women with impaired glucose tolerance is cost-effective," *International Journal of Technology Assessment and Health Care*, Spring 2007; 23(2):177–183.

CHAPTER 8

Why Some Think Threading the Artery Is Easier Than Threading the Needle in Cardiovascular Disease

THE TERM "CARDIOVASCULAR DISEASE" sends a shiver down the spines of many in the Baby Boomer generation. By definition, this term refers to abnormalities in the heart or blood vessels anywhere in the body, but in the United States, it almost always means disease in the arteries that supply blood to the heart or to the brain. And the shiver it causes in many people is a real one, because it affects about 60 million people in this country.[1]

In almost all cases, blood vessel disease is atherosclerosis, often called "hardening of the arteries." We know that atherosclerosis occurs in people with high levels of a certain type of cholesterol, which in turn is affected or amplified by genetics, diet, and level of physical inactivity. Recently, it appears that even recurrent infections of various types during life, such as influenza and gingivitis (gum disease almost always due to chronic infection), are probably also culprit. There is a generalized inflammation in the entire body that come from these infections that, in turn, damages small and medium-sized blood vessels, setting the stage for the early changes of atherosclerosis to begin.

Cardiovascular disease (CVD) is big business as well. Although it is very difficult to get a handle on the costs of all aspects of the treatment of cardiovascular disease, from simple interventions to expensive interventions such as coronary bypass and angioplasty procedures, the use of the latter procedures alone cost well in excess of $250 billion per year in the United States. This is somewhere around 15% of the *entire* health care budget in the most heavily medicalized society in the world.

A very large economics or health policy book would be required to examine the intricacies of CVD care; a single chapter in a general book such as this one can't come close to being comprehensive. But we can ask and answer a straightforward question: "Are we getting our money's worth?" The answer, measured in terms of the increase in longevity and quality of life for the gargantuan sums spent on cardiologists, procedures, hospitalizations, drugs, and complications from all of the interventions, is a resounding *no.* We can also ask, "Can we do better with the money we are spending?" The answer is unequivocally *yes.*

PUTTING A PRICE ON QUALITY OF LIFE

Let's define a few terms to clarify the mind-numbing jargon that physicians and health care planners throw around (often incorrectly). As new information is published in the future, and as political candidates debate the merits of new approaches to "cost-effective" health care, it will be easier to separate the substantive from the fluff.

First and most important is the term "cost-effective." What do economists and insurance companies mean by that term? The cost-effectiveness of a set of interventions or decisions is defined simply as the number of lives saved per dollar spent, or, as it is more usually expressed, as the number of dollars spent to save one year of life.

Consider the level of cost-effectiveness on patients who get vascular surgery due to their dependence on dialysis. Vascular surgery is almost always done on patients who get dialysis to create an easy-to-access and abnormally large vessel—called a shunt—through which blood can be taken and redelivered to the patient. It's expensive (one-time cost of several thousand dollars), and sometimes the shunts become infected or a clot forms in them, requiring additional medical treatments. But even these costs are known, and the probabilities of the complications with shunts or dialysis itself are well-known with exquisite precision. New medications have been developed to prevent some of these complications in the first place.

After years of interviewing patients, the previous unquantifiable "costs" of lost time, mild to moderate discomfort during and shortly after dialysis, and the dietary restrictions that are necessary to avoid the need for *daily* dialysis have been measured, among myriad other impacts on usual activities. These costs aren't typically measured in dollars but rather as decrements from an otherwise healthy, or normal, life, the "quality adjusted life" score we've seen earlier in this book.

The net result is that one can calculate a dollar cost per quality-adjusted life year (QALY). While every physician and layperson recognizes that there is no value one can put on a life, resources are always limited; there isn't even an infinite amount of water or clean air to go around anymore and both are required for life. As a society, we have become comfortable with talking about the "cost per QALY," and the phrase appears in thousands of academic papers every year.

The QALY for dialysis, taking into account surveys from patients on how a year on dialysis compares to a year not having to have dialysis, along with the strictly monetary costs, comes out to about $30,000. This number—which obviously varies somewhat from person to person—is useful for a handful of reasons.

1. First, it provides a measure of what we as individuals and as a society are willing to pay for a procedure that we know from the start is going to go on for years.

2. Second, it provides a benchmark against which other very technology- and time-intensive procedures and services in medicine can be measured. When such comparisons are done, the results are often surprising.

3. Third, think about the health care policy debates that properly occupy more and more of public discourse as the percentage of GDP spent on health care increases. As our population ages, this dialogue is an inevitable result of the demographics already built into the future based on past births, immigration, and changes in death rates from some diseases. From this debate we can get an approximate idea of what we'll need to pay for, which in turn may inform us on how we'll do it. How we'll do it is no small challenge.

Another term that finds its way into almost all discussions of prioritizing health care interventions is "predisease risk." This phrase quantifies, on a scale of 0% to 100%, the probability that a given individual will develop a certain disease based on known risk factors or predictors of that disease. For example, a 25-year-old white, well-educated, urban-dwelling, nonobese female, who has no family history of coronary disease and who does aerobic exercise every day of the year for 20 minutes a day, has a risk of less than 1% of developing coronary artery disease over the next five years of her life.

Contrast this picture of health with a 55-year-old obese, diabetic American Native male who smokes, has high blood pressure, doesn't exercise, and has two brothers in their early sixties who suffered heart attacks at about the age of 55. This poor fellow has about a 50% chance of developing severe symptomatic coronary disease in the next 5 years. (He probably already has advanced atherosclerosis that might not yet have manifested any symptoms other than occasional chest pain when climbing stairs.)

A final key term draws a distinction among the types of prevention: primary and secondary prevention. *Primary prevention* means actions taken *before* disease manifests itself. A simple example is exercising to prevent obesity or high blood pressure. *Second prevention* is intervention once a disease has become manifest (for example, taking high blood pressure medicines once the doctor finds that your blood pressure is elevated).

The distinctions aren't always precise. Taking blood pressure medication can be considered a primary prevention against heart disease because we know that untreated hypertension can caused the heart muscle to thicken and function inefficiently, leading to heart failure or even a stroke or accelerated atherosclerosis.

So, given a risk of developing CVD and the interventions that can prevent or decrease the probability of CVD over a given period of time, we can determine for just about any individual what interventions, if any, should be undertaken to minimize the risk and even calculate the cost of so doing. We can express that cost as dollars per QALY, but remember that the latter already includes the difficult-but-important-to-measure parameters such as inconvenience and side effects.

Then we can go one step further and *rank-order* or *prioritize* the interventions that make the most sense. Finally, we can ask, "Is the American medical system doing the high-priority, cost-effective (or lowest-cost-per-QALY) things it should be doing, or is it squandering money on interventions that are extremely expensive on the QALY scale?"

WHAT INTERVENTIONS ARE AVAILABLE TO PREVENT CVD?

Physicians have about a half dozen choices for medications and life-style modifications that clearly work for both primary and secondary prevention in CVD. They are:

- Advising smokers to stop
- Using of small doses of aspirin (baby aspirin is usually sufficient)
- Treatment of moderately elevated high blood pressure
- Treatment of severely elevated blood pressure
- Treatment of elevated cholesterol

- Use of antiplatelet drugs to prevent coronary clots from forming

With the exception of the last item, most of us are aware of the potential efficacy of each of these intervention in the primary prevention of CVD. After a heart attack (or severe angina warning of the near certainty of heart attack), the same interventions can be used for secondary prevention. Specifically, given that atherosclerosis is clearly established and causing problems, once the pressing complication is taken care of and assuming the patient survives, it is obviously desirable to keep the atherosclerosis from returning. So these same medications are started after a heart attack (unless there is no problem with blood pressure). The antiplatelet drug (usually a medication called Clopidogrel) is new and quite expensive.

Now what are the relative merits of each of these preventative measures, both in the primary context or in the secondary context. Figure 8-1 gives an approximate accounting based on studies in both the British and American medical literature.[2] In calculating the numbers, researchers assume that there is a 10% "baseline" risk of CVD in an individual before primary prevention begins and then a 25% chance of recurrence after a serious event—such as a heart attack or very bad angina symptoms—for the secondary prevention case.

Several things are apparent from this table. First, the higher the risk is, the *lower* the cost is for any intervention to save one year of life (again, quality adjusted). The reason is simple: since more people are at risk, the chances that at least someone in a group of, say, 1,000 people will be helped are higher than if there are few people at risk in that same group. Of course, those people in the secondary prevention group are lucky because they survived their first cardiovascular disease event, when mortality can be high. As but one example: at least 30% of first heart attacks in the United States result in nearly instantaneous death (called "sudden death"). So, all things considered, even though primary prevention appears to be more expensive per life saved, that's largely an artifact of ignoring those poor people who died before getting any primary prevention.

Second, there are huge variations in the benefits from a particular

FIGURE 8-1. The relative merits of preventative measures, both in the primary context or in the secondary context based on studies in both the British and American medical literature.

Intervention	Primary or Secondary or Both	Cost per QALY for Primary Prevention	Cost per QALY for Secondary Prevention
Physician advice for smoking cessation	Both	$ 1,300	$ 4,000
Aspirin	Both	$ 7,000	$ 2,600
Low-intensity high blood pressure treatment	Both, but mostly primary	$ 24,000	$ 9,600
High-intensity high blood pressure treatment	Both, but mostly primary	$ 67,800	$ 27,200
Anti-cholesterol medication	Both	$244,800	$ 98,000
Anti-Platelet drugs	Secondary	$703,000	$421,800
Coronary bypass	Both, but mostly secondary	—	$ 42,500
Coronary angioplasty	Both, but mostly secondary	—	$ 25,000

intervention. Aspirin saves lives at very low cost, even when the potential serious side effects, such as bleeding, are taken into account, but anticholesterol medications are 40 times as expensive on a comparative basis.

Finally, the simplest measure—brief advice to stop smoking in those patients who do—is the most cost-effective of all. Although not every CVD patient smokes, and even though counseling isn't always effective, it is clearly worth the time of the physician and the insurance company that pays for the physician's fee.

To look at this exhibit another way, it is easy to see that:

- For the cost of one coronary bypass procedure, six times as many lives could be saved by prescribing aspirin. At least twice as many lives could be saved by treating moderately elevated blood pressure.

- Taking a cholesterol-lowering medication, easy and attractive as it sounds on television advertisements, isn't very cost-effective at all. Indeed, it is much more expensive per year of life saved than dialysis for patients with renal failure, and most people agree that dialysis is one of the more costly procedures in medicine.

The disparities in benefits are even more stark when visualized as a chart in Figure 8-2, which comes from an independent set of studies[3] that compares cost for QALY via the use of a single high blood pressure medication (called ramipril) and other blood pressure medications in patients with existing CVD with:

- Cholesterol drugs (called "statins")

- Treatment of everyone with mild high blood pressure but not yet with coronary disease

- Angiography and bypass procedures

- In patients with CVD, treatment with a single high blood pressure drug (even if high blood pressure doesn't exist), saves a year of life and the cost of about $2,000 (roughly £1,000).

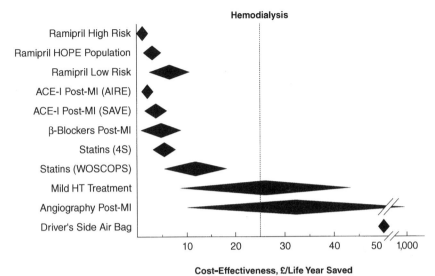

FIGURE 8-2. The disparities in benefits from an independent set of studies comparing cost of QALY via the use of a single high blood pressure medication (called ramipril) and other blood pressure medications in patients with existing CVD.

Like the previous exhibit, this graph teaches several important lessons:

- The use of cholesterol drugs in patients with established CVD is at least four times as expensive.

- Invasive procedures performed by a cardiologist (such as angiography) are very cost-*ineffective* and also have a wide range of uncertainty because the rate of use of procedures like angiography are, as we have already seen, highly variable.

- Compared to dialysis, the simple treatments are very inexpensive, but invasive cardiovascular procedures are not

- And interestingly enough, the driver's side air bag—which is standard on most cars these days—is much more expensive per year of life saved than any of the medical procedures!

So, you'd think we'd do the cost-effective things first, right? But you'd be wrong (as the widespread adoption of driver's side air bags already hints). Here are the sad facts about the treatment and prevention of CVD in America:[4]

- Only about 35% of patients at risk for CVD are taking aspirin (even after eliminating patients who cannot tolerate aspirin for one reason or another). Compared to European countries, only about half as many Americans eligible to receive aspirin for secondary prevention—that is, after an event has taken place—actually get it.

- Physician-owned cardiology specialty hospitals are no better than community hospitals in providing prescriptions for aspirin and beta blockers (another very effective medication for decreasing the likelihood of a second heart attack).

- While cholesterol drug prescriptions have increased dramatically in the past 10 years, physician recommendations to take aspirin have not. In fact, it appears that patients taking cholesterol medications are *less* likely to take aspirin than patients not taking cholesterol medications, suggesting that there is a belief among physicians and/or patients that cholesterol medications are so effective in preventing CVD that aspirin is not necessary. From a cost and effectiveness standpoint, that is precisely incorrect.

For disease closely related to coronary artery atherosclerosis, such as stroke (also called "cerebrovascular disease"), aspirin and treatment of high blood pressure may be even *more* effective in primary prevention of stroke that in primary prevention of heart attack. It is thus tragic that these simple, inexpensive interventions are even less likely to be used for stoke prophylaxis than heart disease prophylaxis.

Commenting on the failure in Britain's national health service to utilize the well-known data of incremental cost-effectiveness of the various strategies just outlined for preventing cardiovascular disease, the *British Medical Journal* editor wrote:

From air travel to patient safety to coronary heart disease prevention, people strive to reduce risk to zero. We know that zero risk is unattainable, yet we pursue perfection. It may be useful to hold perfection as an ideal, but there can be great harm in trying to achieve it because near perfection often imposes near infinite costs. The closer we get to perfect risk reduction, the more likely it becomes that we could have got a better bang for our preventive buck somewhere else. This applies across all activities—and needs to be heeded in health care as anywhere else.

. . . In health care, cost remains something of a dirty word, and including evidence about costs in clinical guidelines remains controversial. But costs are not just cash. Advocates of evidence-based medicine advise doctors to think of costs as "other treatments you can't afford to do if you use your scarce resources to do this one," noting that "when internists borrow a bed from their surgical colleagues in order to admit a medical emergency tonight, the opportunity cost includes tomorrow's cancelled surgery."

. . . Should national guidelines be amended to offer preventive measures in order of incremental cost effectiveness? Absolutely, because any other action guarantees less gain in health for whatever is spent. Across the entire NHS, following the current guidelines would waste billions of pounds and prevent fewer coronary events than if cost effectiveness were used to guide treatment. Evidence based clinical guidance must include incremental cost effectiveness, to prevent the pointless and profligate pursuit of perfection.[5]

The science is clear from many years of research and observation: inexpensive preventative measures are available to forestall CVD that, while far from perfect, are safe and easily affordable, reducing costs dramatically down the road. Yet in the United States our focus—and by far most of the cost—of treating CVD remains in the high-tech procedures and medications that are lucrative to physician specialists and drug companies. Here the value to the patient and to society is the least favorable; as is all too human, physicians and others tend to follow the money instead of the science. In a world of limited resources, and especially in a profession that is supposed to put the interests of patients first and foremost—not only must we do better, it is quite apparent that we can.

And if we don't, costs will continue to rise and more people will lose years of life that could otherwise be lived with happiness in good health.

NOTES

1. *The American Journal of Cardiology*, 2003; 91(suppl): 22G–27G.
2. Jeffrey L. Probstfield, MD, "How cost-effective are new preventive strategies for cardiovascular disease?"*The American Journal of Cardiology*, May 22, 2003; 91(10A): 22G–27G; Tom Marshall, "Coronary heart disease prevention: insights from modeling incremental cost effectiveness," *British Medical Journal*, November 29, 2003; 327: 1136.
3. I. S. Malik, V. K. Bhatia, J. S. Kooner, "Cost effectiveness of ramipiril treatment for cardiovascular risk reduction," *Heart*, 2001; 85: 539–543.
4. Randall S. Stafford, Veronica Monti, and Jun Ma, "Underutilization of aspirin persists in US ambulatory care for the secondary and primary prevention of cardiovascular disease," *PLoS Medicine*, December 2005; 2(12): 1292–1298.
5. Rebecca Warburton, "What do we gain from the sixth coronary heart disease drug?" *British Medical Journal*, 2003; 327: 1237–1238.

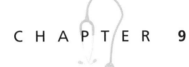

C H A P T E R 9

Degenerative, Infectious, and Autoimmune Diseases

ODD AS IT MAY SEEM, diseases as seemingly different as tuberculosis, rheumatoid arthritis, and the long list of so-called "degenerative" problems such as Alzheimer's or osteoarthritis, are linked. They are all, to one extent or another, affected by the immune system and largely augmented by the immune system's collection of billions of white blood cells, lymph nodes, and dozens of specialized cells that reside practically everywhere. They are also linked by the odd combination of socioeconomics and politics that characterizes much of medicine: the overall misallocation of resources and attention in health care, as illustrated by other specific disease entities we've covered, along with the evidence for systemic problems in healthcare delivery no matter what the disease or specialty.

There have been a very few exciting breakthroughs that get enormous attention and money, yet the simple things that can be done now and that have a large beneficial return don't seem to warrant much attention. For example, in the world of infectious disease treatment we've come up with a few truly amazing new antibiotics against certain bacteria in the past few years, but the overuse of these drugs has led to increased resistance among microbes, complicating the treatment of once easy-to-cure infectious diseases. We have new diagnostic techniques that can identify the presence of organisms in a few hours (or even less) based on isolating and characterizing the genome of those organisms in the laboratory. These techniques enable us to know exactly which infection is afflicting a patient with chronic or severe illness, yet we don't have a simple public health surveillance system in order to know when a common organism—say, a new strain of influenza—is spreading in the population until it's too late to do much about it. There are dozens of experimental trials using stimulants of the body's own immune system to fight infection (though none of them has successfully worked, hope springs eternal, as do big grants from the National Institutes of Health), but we can't get physicians who care for people in hospitals and nursing homes to take a flu shot every year, so that they themselves don't become vectors of disease.

In short, the balkanization of medicine—with each health care provider and hospital or clinic staff exquisitely aware of their small piece of the health care puzzle but little else—has created intense excitement in areas that currently help a few (and *may* turn out to help lots of people). However, the tools at our disposal that work and work cheaply are overlooked ("too boring to think about," as one physician blithely remarked when reminded to get his flu immunization before walking into his local nursing home after seeing coughing patients in his office all day).

In this chapter, we'll review some of the progress and a bit of puffery in the diseases that are intimately and obviously tied to the immune system. Although it's still considered novel to put infectious disease in this category, it is now more or less widely appreciated among researchers and practitioners that successful eradication of an infection requires much more than a drug, even if that drug kills 100%

of organisms in the Petri dish. The immune system must work in concert with medications to eliminate a serious infectious disease in the much more complex environment of the body; so we feel it logical to include infectious disease in our discussion of what's right and what's wrong with the medical system's ministering to immune system problems.

THE FIRST LINE OF DEFENSE

In the skin, the lining of the nose, airway passages, intestinal tract, joints, urinary system and even the nervous system, immune system cells serve as sentinels to detect and counter external threats to the body. Stopping the progression of infection is the most obvious function of the immune system, but it also protects us against toxins accidentally ingested or inspired, and even attempts to eliminate cancer cells that have started to form when the normal process of cell division and replacement goes awry.

A few minutes of thought reveals how remarkable the immune system is. Every minute of every day we come into contact with countless organisms (bacteria, viruses, and the like) when we sit on a park bench, play in the park with the dog, pet the dog, or let the dog lick us in the face. On foods, on innumerable surfaces both in the house and outside, while shaking hands or kissing someone we love, billions of organisms may attach to the skin, mouth, eyes, gastrointestinal tract, or elsewhere on or in the body. Yet, despite the battlefield-in-miniature taking place around the clock everywhere in bodies, we don't notice anything.

Sometimes an infection—say from influenza, a very nasty virus that many people incorrectly confuse with the virus types that cause the common cold—will spread to many cells while the immune system struggles to keep the infection in check. To do that, the immune system has to destroy the cells harboring the virus; there is no other way to get rid of any viruses because they are always located inside some host cell in the lungs or other tissues. As a result, we get "sick," that is, we develop symptoms such as a cough, fever, and generalized aching that are really as much an effect of the immune system itself as they are of the invading organism.

Even more remarkable is that the billions of potent cells that make up the immune system, each empowered to destroy other cells and invading organisms, rarely do any damage to our own tissues. It would be as if an army that is constantly at war over many decades never had a casualty due to "friendly fire." The immune systems in humans, as well as in other mammals, manage to pull off this remarkable feat for our entire lives in almost everyone. Immunologists refer to this as the immune system's "self-recognition" property or, more broadly, as "immune tolerance to self-antigens (proteins)."

But on occasion the immune system fails in one or both of its jobs. Common, usually nondisease-causing organisms can suddenly result in life-threatening infections. And, perhaps less commonly, the immune system can overreact to the presence of a foreign material or organism, leading to organ damage. In fact, it appears that the immune system sometimes does damage to our own organs in the absence of any inciting event such as an infection or injury. Physicians classify the set of diseases described by this last example as the "autoimmune diseases," which will now be reviewed in some detail.

RECENT BREAKTHROUGHS IN UNDERSTANDING THE IMMUNE SYSTEM

The medical discipline or subspecialty that studies and treats immune system disorders is called immunology. The clinical practice of immunology is usually broken down into three groups: (1) allergy (in this subspecialty the physicians are called "allergists"), (2) rheumatology (the physicians are known as "rheumatologists"), and (3) laboratory immunology, which comprises most of the fundamental research into the immune system.

But even this description is incomplete because, as already noted, diseases of just about any organ or organ system involve the immune system to some extent. As but one additional example, almost all of the subset of serious dermatologic conditions are, it appears, due to aberrations in immune system function. The same is true for neurologists who treat debilitating disorders such as multiple sclerosis or Guillane-Barre syndrome, which can lead to paralysis and widespread nervous system failure. (Though it is through different mechanisms, the immune system is clearly involved in the progression of these diseases, and many people believe—with some good evidence—that infection was the inciting event, precipitating immune system overreaction and damage to vital tissues in the process.) So it is probably fair to say that all physicians, no matter what their specialty, are acting as "immunologists" from time to time.

But as recently as the late 1970s, immunology was largely a backwater in medicine. Without the ability to study the internal functions of cells, let alone what we now know to be the enormously complex chemical signaling that takes places among the hundreds of millions of tiny components immune system, the field was simply too mind-boggling to contemplate. Funding from the National Institutes of Health was directed more at finding new antibiotics, treating coronary disease, and coming up with new chemicals to combat cancer.

Then in the early to mid-1980s came reports of a strange disease among mostly homosexual men on the East and West Coasts. Suddenly, otherwise healthy-appearing young men developed previously rarely described infections in their lungs with a protozoa-like organism that was commonly found in soil and thought to have no potential to cause disease. They developed tumors in their skin that appeared as large, purplish blotches on the legs and face. Some became demented or had dangerous infections in their brains at an age in life when such problems almost never occurred. And many went on to die.

As the reports slowly started to accumulate, a name was given to this constellation of bizarre infections and symptoms. The name, Gay-Related Immune Deficiency Syndrome (GRIDS), reflected the belief—which turned out to be true—that a catastrophic failure in the immune system was the underlying reason for the strange (indeed sometimes novel) infections and tumors in these individuals.

Similar case reports came from all over the world, including Europe and the Caribbean. And a few epidemiologists who had worked in central and sub-Saharan Africa noted that the weight loss and muscle wasting that accompanied the other symptoms of GRIDS were reminiscent of a poorly understood malady first described in the 1950s: the "slim disease" of some African populations where young men and women slowly started to lose their appetite and energy levels. They acquired unusually severe cases of tuberculosis or similar infections and went on to die.

The worlds of medicine and the media were alarmed. And because it appeared that GRIDS occurred in not just homosexual men (though they were, by far, the largest segment of the immune system failure syndrome cases identified), another name appeared: the Acquired Immune Deficiency Syndrome (AIDS). The word "acquired" meant a noncongenital cause (that is, acquired during life), with abnormalities in just about any of functions of the immune system that the limited technology of the time could measure.

Of course, we now know the cause: a virus so remarkable that, when its function was first described, even the discoverers could scarcely believe it. The virus is now known as the Human Immunodeficiency Virus, and it is, beyond any doubt, the sole cause of AIDS. Until that time, a virus like HIV, which can quite literally integrate its own genetic material into the genome of a wide variety of cells in the human body, most importantly those of the immune system, and cause a uniformly downward course, had never been described.

There is no overstating the remarkable triumph of modern biology and virology to isolate and identify this virus. It took great courage on the part of the HIV's discoverers to put forward the hypothesis that there existed an entirely new class of viruses. These viruses could subjugate the gene-reproducing functions of normal mammalian cells and force them not only to make millions of copies of a virus that would ultimately overwhelm billions of immune system cells, but also to permanently integrate their peculiar genes into the human genome itself. Few would have even permitted themselves to think broadly enough to entertain this possibility. The description of the life cycle of the AIDS virus was a once-in-a-generation scientific tour de force. It is referred to now as "retrovirus" because its peculiar genomic structure is based on RNA, taught for generations to high school students as well as medical school and graduate school aspirants, as the *product of* DNA.

RNA is the template for *making* DNA that could then insert itself into the DNA of human and other mammalian chromosomes—the prohibited "reversal" of what was previously believed as a fundamental tenet of biology to be a one-way-only process.

The appearance of the disease called AIDS and the discovery of the virus that causes it led to a huge realignment in research funding from national governments all over the world. Suddenly, immunology became the central focal point of research. Though no one could have known it at the time, the exploration into the immune system abnormalities induced by HIV has led to effects in essentially every medical specialty and has, in some way, touched on the treatment of diseases that affect organs once though unrelated to immune system dysfunction. We describe some of those diseases now, along with the remarkable advances that have been made in just the past two decades in treating them. As we shall see, the diagnosis and treatment of these diseases are an unusual example in medicine of physicians now doing more good than harm.

THE AUTOIMMUNE DISEASES

The specialty of rheumatology focuses on the treatment of disorders that until just a few years ago almost inevitably led to the loss of function in the joints, muscles, and sometimes internal organs. The names of at least some of these diseases are probably known to most readers: rheumatoid arthritis, systemic lupus erythematosus ("lupus"), and spondylitis (literally, the inflammation of the spine leading to calcification and complete loss of mobility of the spine). Other diseases, rarer and thus less well-known, are:

- Psoriatic arthritis (severe inflammation and destruction of multiple joints in association with the skin disease psoriasis).

- Scleroderma (literally, "hard skin," but actually a body-wide disease where extra collagen accumulates in many organs leading to their failure and death, usually from kidney, lung or heart dysfunction).

- Polymyositis (inflammation of the muscles with the destruction of muscle cells and replacement with immobile fibrous tissue).

Patients with these diseases not only suffer endless pain and varying degrees of immobility, they also used to suffer with the knowledge that much if not most of the time their symptoms would be relentlessly progressive. Despite the best efforts of rheumatologists, physical therapists, nurses, and special hospitals and clinics devoted to the intensive treatment of these patients—sometimes for years—a wheelchair was the destination that many, perhaps most, patients had to look forward to. Many others died from the complications of their diseases.

There had been a few discoveries that led to hopes that safe and effective treatments were around the corner, only to be dashed by terrible side effects or a merely temporary response. For example, in 1948 Dr. Julian Perry of the Mayo Clinic isolated the naturally occurring hormone called cortisone which, when given to rheumatoid arthritis patients who were literally immobilized from joint inflammation and swelling, resulted in some wheelchair-bound individuals standing and walking.

Word quickly spread and chemists found a way to synthesize the compound, turning it into a practical medication. Little did anyone know that the side effects of cortisone and its derivatives—fluid retention, diabetes, muscle wasting, and hypertension to name but a few—would demote it from "cure" for rheumatoid arthritis to "intermittently useful medication for treatment of painful flares." In addition to having these unpleasant side effects, cortisone is—when given in large doses—a general immune system suppressant. Thus, it reduces the inflammation known to occur (though we don't know why it occurs) in rheumatoid arthritis. Unfortunately, it also makes individuals susceptible to various infections, as might be expected.

But with the revitalization of research in immunology—in no small way due to the scourge of AIDS and the discovery of HIV—a panoply of medications has appeared. Some of them are derived from the "molecular probes" that researchers developed to unravel the complex function of the HIV organism and also the aberrant function of the immune system in AIDS patients. As a result, there are now extremely potent medications that target what we believe to be at least some of the specific immune system irregularities in rheumatoid arthritis, even the once almost untreatable inflammation of psoriatic arthritis and spondylitis. Instead of having to rely on general immune system suppressants (like cortisone), rheumatologists can now selectively manipulate the immune system's overreaction that is doing the damage.

Since the new antiautoimmune system drugs have been around for almost 10 years, and since rheumatoid arthritis in particular is a relatively common illness, it is possible to state with a reasonable degree of certainty the risks and benefits of the most important new class of anti-autoimmune drugs: tumor necrosis factor inhibitors. These drugs were named after a naturally occurring compound called "tumor necrosis factor" (TNF) that was first noticed to kill cancer cells in the Petri dish but that actually turns out to have more wide-ranging effects on the immune system .

These drugs have undergone careful studies done by rheumatologists over a long period of time, along with their slow introduction into the general medical community. These are two desirable characteristics of new drug testing and distribution, and they are very much in distinction to what we've seen with, for example, new cardiology procedures. As a result, the following has been shown:

1. First, twice as many patients achieve nearly complete remission of their arthritis (20% versus 10%) than patients who receive the pre-1990 "standard" therapy for rheumatoid disease, which is an enormous advance for a previously untreatable disease.
2. Second, side effects forcing withdrawal of the new drug are no greater in patients receiving the medication than in patients who do not.
3. Third, withdrawal from (or dissatisfaction with) treatment was much less in patients who receive the TNF inhibitors than those who do not.
4. Fourth, on rare occasions—perhaps 1% to 3% of patients depending on the study one reads—there are very serious complications (primarily infection with tuberculosis), but when

informed of this risk before starting on the drug, the vast majority of patients are willing to accept this small risk even though it may result in fatality or a long course of treatment for infection.

Rheumatologists are not the only specialists who treat autoimmune disease. In gastroenterology practice, there are many patients with a condition known as "inflammatory bowel disease" (IBD), which is really two or three separate diseases that are chronic and painful with often marked disability and impact on daily life. Readers probably know the names of some of the inflammatory bowel diseases: ulcerative colitis and Crohn's disease.

The TNF inhibitor drugs have also been tried in patients with ulcerative colitis, and, while the results aren't as robust as in the treatment of rheumatology conditions, it appears that patients respond quickly and have long lasting remissions as well.

Thus, the introduction of TNF inhibitors is a demonstration that "evidence-based" medicine can serve patients well if this widely uttered but poorly understood process is applied correctly. In the case of TNF inhibitors, the large patient trials, the long-term follow-up (more than just a few months), and the continued monitoring of patients have enabled physicians to do the right thing while minimizing the risk.

But just while TNF has helped hundreds of thousands of patients with autoimmune diseases, the most common of rheumatologic disease—osteoarthritis or degenerative joint disease (DJD), which afflicts tens of millions of people in the United States alone—has, for all intents and purposes, not benefited at all from decades of research. More and more anti-inflammatory drugs enter the marketplace, yet we haven't made a dent in the progressive (albeit slowly progressive) nature of osteoarthritis. In the meantime, a wide variety of surgical procedures have been introduced to try to treat the pain and occasional immobility induced by osteoarthritis. While we'll have more to say about DJD, there is an illustrative example of how more harm than good can be wrought by the failure to use evidence-based research. What applies so well to the use, clinical trials, and careful follow-up of patients taking TNF drugs regrettably has not been applied to the treatments recommended for DJD.

Since there are many joints in the body—any of which can be affected by DJD, from the thumb to the joint where the jaw joins the skull, to hip to knee—we'll pick two examples of medicine gone awry, and once again not with an unusual problem but with a common one.

DO WE REALLY KNEE-D THIS?

The knee joint is much like the hinge of a door: it can flex through a wide range, it can "lock" in a fixed position (full extension of the knee), and it can also fail. The analogy isn't complete because doors are inanimate and knees most certainly are not. Yet the wear and tear on a door's hinge joint that eventually causes it to come loose or break is an indication of the repetitive forces that the hinge—and the knee joint—must maintain.

Covering the surface of the end of the femur (the upper leg. or "thigh." bone) and the top of the tibia (the main bone of the lower leg, or "shin") is cartilage, a glassy appearing, rather hard material brimming with cellular activity. Within the cartilage cap on the bones that make up the knee joint are countless specialized cells—called "chondrocytes"—that continuously make cartilage and remodel the caps of the femur and tibia. Several ligaments—tough, leather-like, ropy connections between bones—are found within the joint and around it. In addition, circular, two silver-dollar–sized disks of cartilage called the menisci are found between femur and tibia. The menisci slide back and forth as the knee bends (and it does so many thousands of times a day and often with substantial pounding thrown in from running, jumping, or even just walking on a concrete surface).

It is amazing enough that the knee's cartilage lasts for a few months under all of this stress, let alone many decades before starting to lose the battle with age or, in the case of some athletes, with absurd levels of abuse. Most readers will be unsurprised that football players who are tackled by 300-pound linemen 50 times every Sunday— usually with a helmet leading the lineman's way—often end up with knee problems. (On average, about one NFL player is carried off the field every week holding his knee in pain after being tackled or catching a football and running into a player even larger than himself.) Like all of the human body, the knee's mechanical design and resilience constitute an engineering marvel.

But for most of us—and not just athletes or professional football players—eventually the cartilage-producing cells within the cartilage itself seem to stop doing their job, or at least slow down so much that the daily accumulation of damage to the cartilage from just normal activity is not fixed. The result is cracks and thinning in the substance of the cartilage. Mensici may become so thin (or subjected to so much force from, say, a sharp turn on the ski slope) that they tear. When those or any of a myriad of other anatomic changes take place, pain occurs, and the cartilage damage may get so bad that there is not much of a protecting cap over the femur or tibia, allowing the bony undersurface of one to rub on the other. Osteoarthritis is, by definition, the diagnosis.

Back in the early 1980s, orthopedic surgeons got the idea that little chips of broken-off cartilage, cracks in the meniscus, and the inflammatory reaction of the body to the degenerative mayhem taking place inside the knee joint might be ameliorated by making a small incision in the knee joint and inserting a fiber-optic instrument called an "arthroscope" to visualize the damage. Then, via the miracles of modern engineering, they could use the same small flexible tube to remove cartilage pieces, wash out the joint with an enzyme-containing cleaning solution, and maybe even remove pieces of menisci that seemed to merely be getting in the way of normal joint function. Thus, the field of arthroscopic knee surgery was born.

By the early 1990s, more than half a million people a year underwent arthroscopic knee surgery at a cost of at least $5,000 each.[1] Many patients were convinced they were helped. The number of surgeons happily willing to do this procedure (pocketing about $2,000 for less than one hour's work) skyrocketed, as did the popularity and number of arthroscopic knee operations for DJD.

But there was a problem: no one had thought to see if the procedure really helped by doing a careful, controlled trial. Such a field test would be difficult to do. For one thing, it was difficult to create a "control" or "placebo" group; that is, a group of patients who *thought* that they had had an arthroscopy, but who really were just put to sleep with a tranquilizer and had small incisions made in the skin of their knee, but did not actually have the knee opened or an arthroscope inserted.

But a creative group of physicians in the Veteran's Administration's hospital system got permission to do just such a trial. One hundred eighty patients with osteoarthritis of the knee were randomly assigned to one of three groups: (1) those who received arthroscopy with removal of joint debris; (2) those who received arthroscopy with washing (or "lavage") of the joint space alone; and (3) the placebo group who had small incisions made in their skin (while under mild anesthesia) while sounds from splashing saline solution permeated the operating room.[2] Outcomes—primarily complaints of pain and satisfaction with functional results—were measured over two years.

The results were surprising, and they continue to generate no small amount of resentment in the orthopedic community: there was no difference in outcome in the three groups at anytime in the two-year follow-up period. The limitation of the study—fully acknowledged by the researchers—was that, since the operations were done in a VA setting, the population was exclusively male, but there is little reason to believe that osteoarthritis in females is substantially different than in males.

The article summarizing the research has been cited 279 times by other articles as of late 2007, some five years after its publication; the average medical or science journal article is cited one or two times before everyone forgets about it. So what's even more impressive is that the "placebo-controlled" arthroscopy article continues to be cited at about the same annual rate now as when it was first published— quite a remarkable record by medical publishing standards.

There has been little refutation of the article, though plenty of angry commentary. One very recent example illustrates the huffiness but also the key problem in much of medicine (and perhaps more so in surgical specialties): the dominance of "opinion" over science.

> What, if any, are the indications for arthroscopic debridement of the osteoarthritic knee? The question is not new. Yet, recent evidence has either meticulously refined or offhandedly misconstrued an answer to this

clinically significant question. Misunderstanding may be based on scientific investigation of patients with diverse study inclusion and exclusion criteria having assorted surgical procedures and being evaluated by varying outcome measures. For example, some investigators study patients with acute mechanical symptoms and mild degenerative disease and others investigate subjects with chronic pain and advanced osteoarthritis. Some define debridement as a combination of lavage and removal of mechanically disturbing tissue debris whereas others aggressively abrade, drill, or excise areas of eburnation or osteophytes. Some measure outcome based on patient satisfaction, relief of pain, or avoidance of joint replacement arthroplasty, while others evaluate subjective or objective knee scores that may or may not be validated for the condition under review. Ultimately, randomized, controlled clinical trials with clearly defined inclusion and exclusion criteria, appropriate arthroscopic techniques, adequate statistical power, and valid, disease-specific outcome measures will answer the question while minimizing study bias.

Pending such investigation, it is the opinion of the authors that arthroscopic debridement is a reliable and effective treatment for knee arthritis in appropriately selected patients.

. . . In summary, indications for arthroscopic debridement of the osteoarthritic knee do exist. Although the ultimate and natural history of the degenerative process may not be altered, decreased knee pain and improvement in function may be expected in carefully selected patients. Patients must be counseled that in addition to the routine risks of knee arthroscopic surgery and anesthesia, the results of arthroscopic debridement of the osteoarthritic knee are not entirely predictable, the goals are limited, and that their prognosis includes a likely need for future and additional arthritis treatment including a possible need for future reconstructive surgery.

In conclusion, we believe our opinions to be well stated and corroborated by the Arthroscopy Association of North America Position Statement on Osteoarthritis: "There is . . . a sub-group of patients with knee arthritis that can be significantly helped with appropriate arthroscopic surgery.[3]

But, since no controlled trials have been done, the authors don't know what the subgroup "that can be significantly helped" is or what the degree of benefit will be. And that's one very big clue as to why medical care costs as much as it does in the United States and why we seem to be reaping little in return.

MAKING A PAIN IN THE NECK EVEN WORSE

DJD can affect the many joints—sometimes also called "articulations"—between the vertebrae in the neck. The neck, more properly known as the cervical spine, is also a remarkable structure. It can pivot, turn, rotate, bend, and stretch—all while holding the 11-pound head and its contents on top—and do so for decades without giving most people the slightest reason to complain. We bump our heads, quickly turn to look for oncoming traffic, look around corners, and bend down hundreds of times a day, and the muscles and joints of the neck perform flawlessly.

But at any given time, there are millions of people who have a sore neck or muscle tension that may be related to stress, a low-speed automobile accident, or any of dozens of other minor traumas that in general don't cause a whiff of trouble but for some reason become incapacitating. On occasion, the spinal cord, which is surrounded by the vertebrae in the neck, can become compressed. Similarly one of the eight pairs of nerves that leave the spinal cord (one each on the left and right sides of each vertebrae) can also be "pinched." The former condition—sometimes but rarely serious—is called "myelopathy" and can result in the loss of function of the nerves that run down the spinal cord all of the way to the legs. The latter condition is called "radiculopathy" and can, on occasion, result in pain in the upper extremities and much less commonly the loss of muscle tone or function in the arms.

Chiropractors, orthopedic and neurosurgeons, primary care doctors, massage therapists, acupuncturists, and homeopathic doctors make much of their living trying to help such patients. We'll focus on the surgeons here because there is troubling data to indicate that, despite a complete absence of evidence to support the practice, surgeons are increasingly offering desperate patients a surgical treatment that can cost between $10,000 and $100,000 *per operation*. The question is, "Does it do more harm than good?"

The short answer is yes. More than 30,000 neck fusions, disk removals, joint space augmentations, "decompressions," and the like were done in the United States last year alone. Neck surgery has replaced surgical procedures on the brain as the most commonly done *neuro*surgical procedure. Orthopedic surgeons have been doing neck surgery with increasing frequency since abandoning routinely operating on the lower back for almost any chronic pain syndrome in the late 1990s. Insurance companies had stopped reimbursing doctors for the operations (and some patients started suing) because there was no evidence that such interventions worked.

And the same remains the case for neck surgery as this book is written. In the era of what is supposed to be "evidence-based medicine," there is no evidence that surgical intervention for most cases of chronic neck pain work, even when the CAT scan shows degenerative arthritis. Part of the reason is that degenerative arthritis, at least as diagnosed by a radiologist, is seen in about 15% of people over the age of 45 *without* any neck complaints at all—a highly "nonspecific" finding (or one that is riddled with "false positives" as discussed in the chapter on screening tests). What the radiologist calls a disease may be nothing more than an incidental finding.

As this discussion implies, neck surgery is expensive, intensive, and fraught with danger. The most common approach in the patient with chronic neck pain is to "fuse" the joints between two (or among more than two) vertebrae on the theory that excessive motion of a particular part of the neck is squeezing nerves or sometimes the spinal cord. The problem is that, if that were the case, most patients would have specific neurologic findings on examination that show that a specific nerve or segment of spinal cord is not functioning properly. But most patients don't, calling into question the very theory on which the fusion operation is based. In a recent review, perhaps the world's most respected expert in spinal surgery, Dr. Edward Benzel of the Cleveland Clinic. put it this way:

> The surgical management of neck and low back pain can be challenging and often is met with mixed results. It should be considered a last resort. In patients who have failed nonsurgical therapy with a discrete anatomic lesion that correlates with the level of the pain, surgical intervention should be considered. Currently, the mainstay of surgical therapy is fu-

sion through a ventral or dorsal approach. Recently introduced procedures, such as disk arthroplasty, hold great promise, but as yet have not shown improved outcomes over spinal fusion."[4]

But, despite this warning, which has been echoed and preceded by countless editorial and conference presentations, the surgeons persist. Not only is relief of pain rarely achieved, there is now evidence that additional harm may take place. If you think about it, since the neck was designed to move in multiple directions, and since we *expect* our necks to move in multiple directions, if a portion of the neck is intentionally fused—immobilized—then other portions of the neck pick up the slack. They are forced to go through wider movement excursion than normal; that means one would expect more stress on the joints and thus an even greater frequency of wear and tear, that is, *more* DJD.

And that is exactly what we are now seeing. Since the "natural experiment" variation in the use of invasive surgical procedures for chronic neck pain is taking place in enormous numbers, we can look to see if problems are *induced* by the surgery. The results would make anyone considering elective neck surgery (that is, for nonlife-threatening or neurologically threatening symptoms) think again.

We now know—but only after many people have suffered the result—that fusion surgery leads to the acceleration of degenerative change in the neck vertebrae joints above and below the point of operation.[5] It is virtually certain that such patients will develop new complications—pain and loss of motion or function of the neck at best, loss of damage to nerves at worst.

As with the knee arthroscopy procedure, physicians continue to do neck surgery when science says, "Wait." Even before the adverse effects of neck spinal surgery were documented in the literature, evidence- and outcomes-oriented researchers were calling for randomized controlled trials, the only way to know if one is doing more harm than good despite the seductive attractiveness of the underlying theory justifying invasive operations.[6]

Unfortunately, such calls for proper science have been ignored. Patients have paid the price in terms of increased suffering. (Although doubtless some have obtained relief, the likely explanation is a placebo effect, even though anyone who has been through such a difficult surgery and has spent months recovering from it would hate to admit that they may have made a mistake in agreeing to it in the first place.) And we've all paid a price through increased insurance premiums.

INFECTION

Pick up almost any newspaper on any given day of the week, and it's likely you'll read about the latest "flesh-eating bacteria" or "germs that are resistant to all antibiotics." And the problem is real enough; organisms that can't be killed by virtually any antibiotic are becoming more and more common, almost certainly due to the overuse of antibiotics when they are not required or using the wrong antibiotic. It may also be the case that the occasional—but headline-grabbing—cases of fatal infection from ordinary skin organisms due to gangrenous necrosis of the skin and muscle (medicalese for "flesh-eating") are related to antibiotic overuse as well. This is because other organisms that complete with the flesh-eating bacteria are killed by antibiotics, giving these otherwise very rare strains of ubiquitous skin organisms a chance to flourish and, well, eat flesh as well.

Lost in all of the hysteria over these serious but extremely rare infections are the dramatic successes in the prevention of infectious disease, due largely to our increased understanding of how to use and manipulate the human immune system. Vaccinations, once prone to side effects and limited to only a few diseases, are the major manifestations of those successes. The following diseases are now essentially completely preventable with vaccines introduced in the past ten to twenty years:

1. Hepatitis B, once the largest single cause of both chronic liver failure and cirrhosis.
2. Pneumococcal pneumonia—of two dozen subtypes—once the largest cause of bacterial pneumonia.
3. Hemophillus influenza—which actually has nothing to do with the viral disease we now call "influenza"—but is instead a bac-

teria that was once the largest cause of meningitis and subsequent serious developmental delay and neurologic damage in infants and children.

4. And finally, influenza, the leading cause of respiratory disease deaths due to infectious disease in the U.S. and much of the rest of the world.

These vaccines are essentially without side effects, are affordable, and are available everywhere. The only problem remains getting people to take them. Most worrisome and embarrassing is that fewer than one-third of physicians (and only a slightly larger fraction of nurses, nurse practitioners, and other care providers) get an influenza vaccine. In addition to putting themselves at risk for acquiring a very serious infection from the patients they treat, these health care providers become vectors for influenza because the vaccine not only largely prevents disease but when infectious occurs the vaccine dramatically lowers the shedding of virus particles. There is no excuse for this shabby behavior on the part of doctors and nurses. One infected health care provider can infect an entire nursing home or dozens of patients in hospital.

But—bad behavior on the part of health care providers aside—the advances in vaccinology (the science of vaccines) have resulted in a reduction not only of acute fatal disease such as meningitis and pneumonia, but also long-term suffering from a once ubiquitous liver-destroying virus.

As our knowledge of the human immune system continues to advance, more vaccines are in the offing.

At the same time, treatment for AIDS, whose recognition probably did more to advance our knowledge of the immune system than any other single event, has also advanced dramatically. Although not "curable" in the sense of eradicating the HIV organism from an infected individual, AIDS is now a manageable chronic disease. People with AIDS have the reasonable expectation of living for decades after diagnosis when only 10 years ago the infection was fatal to almost everyone within months to a few years after the diagnosis was made.

But other news in the management of infectious disease remains decidedly mixed. There is still no national or even regional disease surveillance and reporting system in the United States, despite the example of such a system in Texas that has been in use for five years by physicians, nurses, veterinarians, and public health officials, and which costs a few pennies per capita per year.[7] Despite this clear success, the U.S. government agencies responsible for protecting the public and the agricultural industry against both naturally occurring disease and the threat of bioterrorism remain intransigent in their resistance to change, employing paper-based reporting systems that have repeatedly failed, costing many lives and hundreds of millions of dollars in agricultural losses. It is long past the time for the proven, inexpensive real-time human and animal electronic reporting system to be put into place.

Physicians continue to overprescribe antibiotics—using drugs designed to treat bacterial infections for the treatment of viral infections. It is estimated that more than 50% of all antibiotic prescriptions written in the United States are either unnecessary or incorrect. The result—multiple strains of bacteria resistant to almost all antibiotics—continues to grow. It is essential that oversight and review organizations find a way to provide incentives to physicians to stop this sloppy, dangerous practice.

Thus, in the world of infectious disease, the picture is ambiguous: dramatic advances in the prevention of the most common lethal infections that are underutilized; the overuse of powerful antibiotics in the wrong circumstances; and a failure to install a desktop electronic disease reporting system via the public health system in the United States to recognize the first cases of both novel diseases (like SARS) or new versions of old diseases (like influenza), so that cost-effective control measures can be put into place before disease spreads. Unless and until the latter is done, we'll be left with the much more expensive, far less effective option of treating sick individuals with the attendant loss of life and also productivity.

MORE ON DEGENERATIVE DISEASE

The usual definition for "degenerative diseases" goes something like this: the dysfunction or change in structure of one or a group of organs that progressively worsens over time. Leading examples are Alzheimer's disease, osteoarthritis [degenerative joint disease (DJD)], and osteoporosis.

Implicit in the definition is that the diseases are somehow related to aging, and, while the association is doubtless, there is nothing inevitable about these diseases occurring with age. Everyone eventually dies, of course, but many people in their eighties and nineties are free of dementia, joint pain, and brittle bones. What accounts for the variation in incidence of "degenerative" problems?

It turns out that many of the diseases we thought of just part of aging or "wear and tear" are, at least in part, due to some impairment in the immune system. For example, in Alzheimer's disease specialized immune system cells found only in the brain—called microglial cells—appear to be overly reactive to the presence of certain proteins that tend to accumulate in the brain with age. In "cleaning up" these proteins, the microglial cells seem to do damage to normal neurons that are the basic cellular units carrying out memory and judgment, and defining personality traits, all of which we know to be clearly damaged in Alzheimer's disease. In experimental animals whose brains undergo the same pathological changes as seen in humans with Alzheimer's disease, immunization against the age-related protein accumulations stop the changes from occurring, strongly indicating that immune system manipulation may hold the key to preventing the progression of the earliest symptoms of Alzheimer's disease or may obviate the disease entirely. In other dementing diseases, the same promise may hold.

And even osteoporosis, "thinning of the bones," is accelerated by certain abnormalities of the immune system. The very drugs that are now used to treat osteoporosis and that were developed with the belief that they worked strictly on the cells creating new bone turn out to be potent immune system stimulants as well.

Thus, in what has to be one of the most unexpected linkages among diseases, infection, degenerative disease of brain, bone, and joints and the autoimmune diseases all are exquisitely dependent on immune system function. It is a triumph of medical research that this recognition has taken place, opening a window based on our ever deepening understanding of the immune system for therapies that have been as successful as those for previously untreatable rheumatoid arthritis and preventative techniques once believed impossible.

All of this was made possible by the careful application of laboratory science in careful, well designed controlled trials, the very essence of the scientific method that has been lacking in much of the rest of medicine. In this important collection of unexpectedly related diseases, the medical system can claim to be doing more good than harm in a few circumstances. But in most cases the story remains the same as in much of the rest of medicine: individual physician "opinion" dominates what we know, and what we don't know, from the evidence.

NOTES

1. J. B. Moseley, K. O'Malley, et al., "A controlled trial of arthroscopic surgery for osteoarthritis of the knee," *New England Journal of Medicine*, 2002; 347(2):, 81–88.
2. The ethical debate of so-called "sham" surgery in the setting of clinical trials received a huge boost from this study, and there is no limit to the number of legitimate questions that can be raised. The ethical considerations could well occupy an entire book; so they shall be conveniently ignored in this chapter.
3. J. Michael, M. D. Stuart, and James H. Lubowitz, M.D., "What, if any, are the indications for arthroscopic debridement of the osteoarthritic knee?" *Arthroscopy: The Journal of Arthroscopic & Related Surgery*, March 2006; 22(3): 238–239
4. Edward C. Benzel et al., "Surgical management of neck and low back pain," *Neurology Clinician,*2007; 25: 507–522.
5. J. T. Robertson, et al., "Assessment of adjacent-segment disease in patients treated with cervical fusion or arthroplasty: a prospective 2-year study," *Journal of Neurosurgical Spine*, 2005; 3: 417–423.
6. Ioannis P. Fouyas, Ph.D., Patrick F. X. Statham, FRCS (SN), and Peter A. G. Sandercock, "Cochrane review on the role of surgery in cervical spondylotic radiculomyelopathy," *Spine*, 27(7): 736–747.
7. Alan P. Zelicoff, M.D., and Michael Bellomo, "A New Weapon in the Fight," in *Microbe: Are We Ready for the Next Plague?* (New York: AMACOM, 2005).

CHAPTER 10

Making the Best Medical Decisions for You

PERHAPS THE MOST PERPLEXING—and unexpected—problem that we've been forced to confront in recent medical history is that mass numbers of people are now living beyond what some scientists refer to as "the design life of the human body," which is roughly 45 to 50 years. Because of this, we've been forced to confront a slew of chronic degenerative diseases for which precious few interventions make much difference. Some of these interventions may prolong life, but often at the cost of much increased morbidity or suffering. And so the questions then become:

- "What preventative measures can you take to ensure the maximum life span for the human body?"

- "How does the wise health care consumer extract the utmost from a health care system that often gives questionable advice and recommends treatments that may benefit someone other than the patient?"

Because we believe the information in this book shows the overwhelming benefits of prevention of disease rather than treatment thereof—even in the 21st century.

THE "ALL YOU SHOULD EAT" SPECIAL

The first part of the answer to extending the life span of the body is everyone's clear favorite: diet. How do we come to this conclusion? Well, just look in the bookstores. There's the South Beach Diet, there's the California Beach Boys Diet; there are diets that indicate we should eat all meat, diets that indicate we should eat no meat, and diets that tell us that if you're not a vegan you're going to die at the age of 40.

But when all is said and done, the major lessons with regard to diet are not so much what you should *avoid* in your diet, such as "simple" carbohydrates (sugary sweets, soft drinks) and fats, but what you *should* include in your diet, independent of whatever else you eat. And while it's not a negligible health matter to be obese, it's better to be a bit overweight and have the right diet than to be thin and have the wrong diet. What is needed is a diet supplying a few nutrients that we now know make a big difference with regard to the big killers out there, coronary disease and cancer being the leading ones. We review the limited, but demonstrably beneficial dietary "inputs" below.

We do need to serve up one disclaimer, however. For many diseases that occur at a low to moderate level—neurological degenerative disease, multiple sclerosis, some forms of rare cancers—there simply isn't enough data to say whether diet makes any difference whatsoever. But because certain cancers, like colon, prostate, or breast cancer, are very common. And certain arterial diseases such as coronary artery disease are also very common. So we now have a large enough data set to indicate what in a diet can make a difference in terms of staving off the likelihood of these diseases.

Even doctors tend to focus on what to eliminate from their diet, though it turns out that it's much more important to focus on what you should be sure to include your diet on a regular basis, independent of everything else. Now, we're not here to argue that it's a good idea to put something good into your diet and then eat a box of snack cakes or to ladle on the bacon grease. But we are here to state that if you're going to do anything at all, it's much better to focus on what to put into your diet than on what to take out.

OILS FROM THE SEA AND THE TREE

With regard to coronary artery disease and also with regard to some cancers, we've now learned that certain types of oils primarily found in deep sea fish have a strong preventive effect. What's more, fish oil is a very cost-effective vehicle for reducing the risk of coronary disease and colon cancer. In the case of breast-feeding women, it appears that fish oil helps in the neurological development of their child. Fish really can be thought of as "brain food"—and, if you don't like fish, you can take the oils in capsule form. The amount of fish we're talking about is 3 and 6 ounces on average a week of deep sea fish: salmon, mackerel, halibut, sardines, anchovies, or tuna. A capsule of fish oil or two a day—the brands don't matter much—are an extraordinarily cost-effective insurance policy against multiple vascular and degenerative diseases. Nothing is 100% guaranteed, of course, but this choice is about as clear as choices get. Here's some of the evidence.

For reasons that we don't fully understand, but probably having to do with reducing the total body burden of inflammation, these fish oils reduce the inflammation that sets up the blood vessels to develop atherosclerosis.[1] This happens primarily in the heart and in the carotid arteries but, for probably quite unrelated reasons, reduces the incidents of colon polyps as well.

Fish oil also appears to have a modest effect on blood pressure, and it appears to lower the levels of "bad" low-density forms of cholesterol while augmenting (or at least not reducing) the levels of "good," or high-density, cholesterol. High-density cholesterol is also raised as a direct effect of exercise, and probably accounts for many of the vascular health benefits of exercise. Fish oils also affect the "toxic" free fatty acids that float around in the blood, such as trans fats from butter and all the things that make wonderful donuts and cakes. The trans fatty acids have a propensity to be what is called "oxidizing," which is a misleading term in chemistry (because oxygen is not always involved), but it refers to the ability to form hard-to-break chemical bonds with surface constituents or perhaps other internal constituents of the lining cells of blood vessels. The oxidation process alters normal proteins and other molecules in delicate blood vessel cells, starting the process of atherosclerosis and maybe even stimulating the immune system to attack the "altered" normal proteins and cause cell damage and death—further amplifying atherosclerosis.[2]

What fish oil seems to do is to decrease the propensity of oxidation to take place. Oxidation can really be thought very much as the first order of aging or degradation of material, much like rust is the degradation of steel—which does in this case involve oxygen. Oxidation in general means stealing electrons from one molecule and using them to form an abnormal bond to another molecule, creating a new chemical compound. The resulting novel compound may be toxic to the local metabolic environment, particularly of the lining of blood vessel cells.

A few other items that we know are important to include in the diet are also complex oils or fatty acids, primarily those from nuts, such as walnuts, almonds, or pecans—but not so much from peanuts. These, too, have been shown to dramatically reduce the likelihood of coronary artery disease, and, in those people who have had treated coronary artery disease, they decrease the recurrence of coronary disease. So, in both a primary preventative setting and in what physicians refer to as a secondary preventative setting (after the disease has become established and then treated), certain nut oils, primarily from walnuts and closely similar nuts, do reduce the likelihood of coronary disease or its recurrence.

Now at this juncture it's important to comment on the use of some vitamins specifically for the prevention of coronary artery disease.

What has grabbed headline attention in the past 10 years or so has been primarily vitamin E. We now know that—after very carefully gathered controlled trials, both in patients at risk for coronary disease because of family history, high blood pressure, and/or high cholesterol, or in those who have already had coronary disease and have undergone therapeutic procedures to remove or byass obstructions in the coronary arteries—vitamin E is largely a waste of money.

Vitamin E also comes with a couple of issues that consumers should be aware of. One of the complications of E comes from the accumulation of large amounts of vitamin E in the body, because it is a fat-soluble vitamin. This means that, unlike the B vitamins or vitamin C, which are soluble in water, vitamin E taken in huge doses does not pass out through the urine. Also, there is a pervasive believe that, "If some is good, more is better." That's a deadly conclusion with vitamin E, because, in high doses, vitamin E can actually be toxic. So there's no evidence to indicate that it is cost-effective to spend your money on vitamin E tablets, but that fish oil tablets, which are cheap and easily available in any food or grocery store are helpful.[3] Small doses of vitamin E [the dose for the fat-soluble vitamins is usually expressed in international units (IU)] in the range of 400 IU is fine, but you'd get that much for a diet that includes dark green vegetables on a daily basis and an avacado every once in a while.

Now, what about problems with fish oil? One concern many people have is that, by increasing your intake of deep sea fish, you could be increasing your intake of mercury and other heavy metals that tend to be concentrated in ocean fish in particular. The short answer is, yes, you likely are going to get larger amounts of trace heavy metals, but even in the case of much-larger-than-average intakes of either fish or fish oil, the benefits strongly outweigh the risks.[4] Even in childbearing women whose legitimate concern is about the effects of mercury on the neurological development of the fetus, moderate (two to three servings per week or a fish oil tablet or two daily) provides more benefit than danger to the fetus.

Finally, the risks of exposure to environmental toxins with fish consumption are substantially reduced through purification processes used to develop selected concentrated fish oil supplement preparations.

So, while fish from areas of the world with high mercury levels in the water have a small, theoretical risk (especially to the developing fetus of a pregnant woman who consumes the fish), the production of fish oil tablets largely eliminates even this very small concern.[5]

ALL THAT IS SWEET ISN'T GOOD

People often ask about sugar and simple carbohydrates in the diet. Simple carbohydrates are nothing more than sugars that occur as either single molecules or maybe two linked molecules of sugar. It's important to understand that a starch, such as in pasta or in bread, is in fact thousands or millions of linked sugar molecules (technically, a "polymer" of sugar molecules from the chemist's perspective). From the viewpoint of the body's digestive processes, they're in very long chains that are not instantaneously absorbed as a tangle of single sugar molecules. The difference between consuming complex carbohydrates—that is, those with countless sugars linked together—versus simple carbohydrates is becoming clear. Although it's somewhat hard to prove (simply because effects accumulate slowly and thus individals have to be observed for very long periods of time, often decades), there does appear to be increasing evidence that consuming simple sugars or carbohydrates (such as what you might find in a soft drink) comes with at least two adverse effects. The first fact to bear in mind is that these sugars rarely result in satiety—that is, the satisfaction that you've consumed enough. And we don't really understand the feedback effect of satiety on the brain from simple sugars well enough to understand why that's the case. So, if you eat 100 calories or 200 calories of pure sugar from drinking a soft drink versus eating two slices of bread that have roughly 200 calories in them, the calorie numbers are the same. But you are far more likely to experience the sensation of fullness from eating the bread than you are from drinking an equivalent number of calories of simple sugars, even if you ingest them over roughly the same period of time, let's say 15 to 20 minutes. Part of it, of course, has to do with the fact that the bulk stretches receptors in the stomach that sends a signal to the brain that one's full. But that's not the complete explanation.

There is now a very recent study that proves what many nutritionists and diabetes experts have long suspected: increased simple sugar intake in the form of sweetened beverages is strongly associated with Type II diabetes in adults.[6]

The other adverse effect is that, even though the total caloric content of two slices of bread is roughly equivalent to the caloric content of a 12-ounce non-diet soda, the absorption rates of the simple sugars is much, much faster than the absorption rate of a starch. That's because a starch has to be broken down by enzymes in the gastrointestinal tract before it can pass across the membranes of the cells in the gastrointestinal tract to get absorbed. The rise in actual glucose content of the blood is naturally moderated by this digestive processes.

But you get a bigger pulse, a more rapid rise. of blood sugar, even if you're not suffering from some dysfunction of your pancreas, after swallowing a sugary drink than you do eating the same amount of calories in the starch. And this *may* be associated with the burn-out phenomenon in the pancreas that seems to characterize the most prevalent type of diabetes, Type II, where the pancreas cells that respond to blood sugar simply become less responsive to wide swings in the blood sugar as a result of the consumption of sugary substances.

So from a statistical standpoint one can correlate the rise in diabetes very closely with the rise in the total consumption of sugary drinks. What appears to explain it is that, if you saturate the glucose susceptors on the pancreatic cells or on other cells across the body, they simply become less numerous or less responsive to rises in glucose, which leads to a slow, progressive rise in the average blood sugar. In the initial stages, people may actually suffer from periods of relatively low blood sugar (so-called "functional hypoglycemia") due to the ingestion of sugary substances. But this is much less common in a teenager than it is in a 20-year-old and even less so in a 30- to 40-year-old.

It may well be that the middle afternoon fatigue that many of us in our fifties and sixties begin to feel is a result of a relative hypoglycemic episode simply because our pancreas is trying to deal with an enormous sugar load that may have occurred as a result of drinking a soft drink or two at lunch. In younger people there are compensatory mechanisms with another hormone called glucagon, which compensates for hypoglycemia or reduced levels of the blood sugar, and that glucagon response goes away as we get older.

Glucagon causes the liver to release stored sugar; its effect is sort of the opposite to that of insulin, which forces liver cells to take up glucose. So you can think of glucagon as a sort of an anti-insulin hormone. It's located in the pancreas and also in the small intestine, but the glucagon response seems to just—for lack of a better phrase—wear off.

Thus, there now appears to be good evidence that sudden swings in blood sugar—or sudden releases of insulin to help the body store that sugar—are associated with higher incidences of diabetes. What remains to be shown—even though common sense would seem to apply—is that the elimination of simple sugars and replacing those calories with complex carbohydrates does indeed *lower* the ever increasing incidence of diabetes in the population. At the moment, prudence would dictate that simple sugars should make up a very small percentage of the calories we consume and that soft drinks containing glucose or fructose (a closely related simple carbohydrate) may do more harm than providing "empty" calories; the recurrent massive sugar loading from consuming may, over the long run, induce diabetes in adults.

A HARD LOOK AT SUPPLEMENTS

Next to the diet question, the most common one is, "Should I take a vitamin supplement?" Well, if you live on 2-liter bottles of cola and potato chips, the answer is yes. But actual vitamin deficiencies are very rare. Despite the many claims of people who believe that megavitamin doses do something other than create very expensive urine, vitamin deficiencies in a diet that is reasonably composed of vegetables, protein-rich plants, and some meat are virtually unheard of in the Western world.

It was relatively common in the 1800s to see people from the

United States or Western Europe who had vitamin C deficiency diseases. That was because vitamin C is generally found only in citrus fruits, which were difficult to obtain for long portions of the year and which, as a water-soluble vitamin, is not stored in the body for very long periods of time. Even today, it's possible to see some vitamin deficiencies in alcoholics. That's because some alcoholics live off of alcohol alone, which gets converted into fat and sugar and makes a perfectly good fuel, albeit not a good fuel to the exclusion of everything else.

But actual vitamin deficiencies are extraordinarily rare in the United States. There are only two exceptions: the lack of adequate iron intake (1) in women who are menstruating and (2) among poor people who may have a diet that is low in meat. Meat contains not just iron, but rather iron complexed with a molecule called hemoglobin, the major constituent of blood and heme, which is the central molecule of hemoglobin and which allows the iron to be absorbed very easily. Taking iron supplements, though beneficial, is not nearly as good from a pure iron absorption standpoint as having meat and heme in the diet. But given that many of us are moving away from the meat-rich diet, particularly in women of reproductive age who are menstruating, iron deficiency is not at all uncommon. Iron supplementation is easy and inexpensive (but also easily overdone in children, so seek advice from a pediatrician where children's diets are concerned).

AN ASPIRIN A DAY . . .

Worth a final mention are still ever increasing discoveries and miracles of low-dose aspirin. It appears to be unequivocally the case that, certainly for secondary prevention and almost certainly for primary prevention (at least in males), low dose aspirin a couple of times a week or daily (a baby aspirin a day, approximately 65 milligrams) is extraordinarily beneficial for the prevention of coronary disease. The only caveat in any of this is for people who have high blood pressure and who therefore have a propensity for strokes. Aspirin does increase the likelihood of a typical nonbleeding stroke's converting to a hemorrhagic stroke in people who take aspirin on a regular basis (and, as we've previously discussed, the outcome from hemorrhagic strokes is, in general, much worse than nonhemorrhagic strokes). So if you're hypertensive, you may not wish to take aspirin, at least until your blood pressure is under control.

THE WAGES OF SWEAT

In the 1970s, the famous marathon runner, Jim Fixx died at the age of 52 of a massive heart attack after his daily run on Route 15 in Hardwick, Vermont. The autopsy revealed that atherosclerosis had blocked one coronary artery 95%, a second 85%, and a third 50%. When this was revealed at the time of his autopsy, people began to debate the relative merits of exercise.

While the effect of exercise on all disease is not known, we have a pretty good idea of the effect of exercise on the most common conditions already outlined in this book, which are diseases of the blood vessels and cancer. We'll review some of the conclusions from controlled trials, but the message from the few carefully done controlled trials on the role of exercise boils down to this: regular three or four days a week), moderate (45 minutes of walking) exercise improves the ratio of muscle to fat and reduces risk factors for cardiovascular disease and probably diabetes as well. When combined with dietary modification—especially, as emphasized earlier, *adding* fish oil to the diet—one can get multiple benefits with very little investment of time.[7] So, unless you are training for an athletic event, the vast majority of benefits from exercise comes with the first small increment of activity.

We know that obesity is associated with an increased risk of cancer, heart disease, and diabetes. Additionally, there is no question that a regimen of 30 minutes of walking per day or 45 minutes 3 or 4 times a week—such that your oxygen consumption level, which is a rough measure of how much fuel you are burning, is about double what it is for resting. Without putting too precise a measure on it, walking should be considered the activity to which one devotes oneself. While it is a great idea obviously to supplement that exercise with a walk with the dog or other pet, pets tend to slow most people down, so note your walking rate, which should cover a mile in about 12 to 15 minutes.

The current recommendations conclude that 30 to 40 minutes a day of regular walking exercise is sufficient to prevent the side effects of being slightly overweight and to prevent you from becoming more overweight. On the other hand, if you're truly obese, having a body mass index of 30 or more (we explain body mass index in a minute), it's probably necessary to increase your activity to about 60 minutes a day at least five days a week. Again, you don't have to be sprinting, but walking 3 to 5 miles per hour over that period will lead not only to health benefits but also to weight loss.

Individuals often ask, "What is an ideal body weight?" But what all adults should really ask themselves is, "What is an ideal body weight for my particular height?" And there is an easy way to calculate ideal body weight, called the "body mass index" or BMI for short. Here's how:

1. Take your body weight in pounds and divide it by 2.2 to convert it to kilograms. Write that number down.
2. Then take your height in inches and divide by 39.4 to convert to meters. (There are 39.37 inches in a meter; don't ask where all of the odd ways of measuring length come from; that's another book!) Write that number down.
3. Next multiply the second number by itself (or "square it" as the math teacher used to say").
4. Finally, divide the last number into your weight as expressed in kilograms.

The ideal BMI is 19 to 25 (and the units for those who are mathematical purists, are kilograms per square meter)—a little toward the lower side for females, a bit toward the upper side for males.[8] Let's take an example (and it's obviously easy to program this into a spreadsheet if you know how to use one, but paper, pencil, and calculator work just fine). Say you are 5 feet 8 inches tall (60 inches) and weigh 170 pounds. Let's go through the arithmetic:

1. Divide 170 pounds by 2.2: about 77.3. We'll call this result A.
2. Divide 68 inches by 39.4: 1.73. We'll call this result B.
3. Multiply B by itself (or B squared): 1.73 × 1.73: 2.98. This is result C.
4. Finally, divide result A by C: 77.3 ÷ 2.98: 25.91.

So this individual would be considered mildly overweight. Obesity kicks in at a BMI of 27–28, and morbidly obese—indicating that a dramatic reduction in life span is going to be dramatically reduced, is, in general, regarded as associated with being 90 to 100 pounds over your ideal body weight given your height. To be a bit more precise, most physicians think of a BMI of 35 as very dangerous if that individual also happens to have high blood pressure or diabetes. Just about every doctor starts to panic if the BMI is 40, whether or not such a very obese individual has any other measureable "risk factors" for shortened life expectancy—primarily high blood pressure or high blood sugar measurements. Needless to say, high BMI levels put a stress on joints.[9]

We all see obesity just by walking down the street (or maybe by sitting down at a fast food restaurant). Obesity is common from the medical perspective. A 5-foot-4-inch female is obese if her weight is 155 pounds, and for males just a few pounds more.

So, if your goal is to bring your body weight down into the ideal range somewhere between 18 and 25 kilograms per meter squared as measured by the body mass index, you'll probably need something close to 60 minutes a day of exercise to start to lose weight. Once you achieve it, you can back off to 30 or 45 minutes a day three to four times a week.

Now, we've just covered the essential basic exercise recommendations, where you get essentially 80% of the life extension benefits that you would otherwise get if you were trained to be an athlete—all by doing rather modest exercise. A somewhat more exacting—and slightly more beneficial—goal is to exercise vigorously enough to get your heart rate up to about 70% of its theoretical peak and keep it there for 30 minutes or so a day. It turns out that maximum or peak heart rate in patients *without* heart disease (a caveat we'll detail a bit more) is inversely related to age. A good rule of thumb is that your maximum, safe heart rate (before irregular heartbeats start to appear in all but well-trained athletes) is 220 minus your age. So, if you are a typical out-of-shape "weekend athlete" at the age of 45 and you'd like to achieve excellent cardiovascular fitness, improve muscle tone, lose fat, and prolong life by decreasing your blood pressure and blood sugar, get your heart rate up to 70% or so of its peak for 30 minutes or so a day. For the 45-year-old:

- The theoretical maximum safe heart rate is $220 - 45 = 175$.

- Beats per minute are $175 \times 70\% = 123$ (or 30 beats if you count your pulse for 15 seconds—which is a quarter of a minute).

Now for the important caveat: most people who haven't done much in the way of exercise for a while—even if they are rather young and even if they have no obvious obesity or known high blood pressure—probably should have a talk with their primary care doctor before doing any of this. No formal cardiac stress test is required in the overwhelming percentage of people, but a careful interview and exam conducted by your family doctor can avoid the small but appreciable risk of diving into exercise too quickly. And everyone who has had some cardiovascular "event"—such as heart attack, angina, or stroke—should begin exercise under a supervised program.

ADDITIONAL BENEFITS OF EXERCISE

Although you can achieve an exercise by walking, biking, or swimming, most people find walking to be the most convenient. Walk five times a week for 30 minutes, achieving a maximal heart rate of about 70% of your maximal heart rate, and you will within a few weeks to months meet the somewhat stringent requirements of the American College of Sports Medicine for so-called cardiorespiratory fitness. This is distinct from managing your weight, but it can give you the buffer that you may need should you be placed in a stress condition—an automobile accident, the need to rescue somebody, perhaps to dash across the street to catch a bus without suffering from a heart attack.

Besides stopping or reversing weight gain, as well as lowering blood pressure and blood sugar, controlled studies—not someone's opinion, but actual experiments with humans—has shown that exercise:

1. Prevents or dramatically delays osteoporosis and muscle atrophy. Obviously, the upper extremities are not exercised very much by walking. We now know that muscle atrophy in the upper extremities is associated independently with a small but measurable increased risk of both mortality as well as quality of life. So, one's ability, for example, to provide self-care is (as we get past the age of 65 or 70) dramatically affected by muscle tone in the upper extremities.
2. Treats anxiety and depression.[10]
3. Relieves many of the symptoms of chronic fatigue syndrome and/or fibromyalgia, a very uncomfortable and extremely difficult-to-treat condition.[11]
4. Improves joint function—up to a point—in patients with common degenerative arthritis (osteoarthritis).[12]

So minimal activity, along with minimal weight training with light weights at home three times a week in the upper extremities, such as lifting light weights over the head or pushups, is more than sufficient for maintaining functionality. And with regard to lower extremity osteoporosis (weakening of the bones), there is good evidence that weight-bearing exercise, walking, or biking is superior to swimming alone. But, in the end, "do the exercise you enjoy" is probably the best advice.

To summarize, our 25 years of research in the area of exercise has left us with a rather simple set of conclusions. There is a law of diminishing returns for the prevention of weight gain, diabetes, and cardiovascular disease. The greatest benefit can easily be maximized for the amount of time invested simply given by achieving about 70% of your peak heart rate five times a week for 30 minutes if you're not overweight, or for 60 minutes if you are until you become normal weight.

(And you will regain your normal weight if you pursue the latter for several weeks to several months.)

BUT DOCTOR, WHY IS MY ATTEMPT AT
WEIGHT LOSS TAKING SO LONG?

People are often frustrated by the fact that it takes a long time to lose weight, and that's because fat is an extraordinarily efficient means of storing energy. One kilogram of fat (about 2 pounds) contains approximately 9,000 calories of energy. So, if you're 20 pounds overweight, you have to get rid of 90,000 extra calories. Yikes! Brisk walking burns up perhaps 300 calories per hour, so getting rid of 90,000 calories made up of stored fat means 300 hours of walking. Even if you walk 5 hours a week, expect that it will take roughly a year to drop 20 pounds of fat. Indeed, this is the basis of the guidance that most physicians give patients who are serious about losing weight in a methodical, sustainable way: don't expect to lose more than about half a pound per week.

Inevitably, some people are desperate enough to lose weight that they ask about medications, like caffeine or ephedrine, pseudoephedrine (no longer easily available over the counter because it can be used to synthesize methamphetamines), or "diet pills" (which in fact *are* amphetamines or closely related to them), to increase the body's basic metabolic rate, consuming calories in the process. While there is always the possibility that some miracle drug capable of doing this safely is just around the corner (and would certain bring huge income to the pharmaceutical company that markets it), the past two decades are littered with failed trials of diet drugs. For all intents and purposes, all such drugs have been taken off of the market because of side effects: constricting blood vessels and thereby increasing the risk of high blood pressure and stroke, damaging heart valves, and causing heart attacks.[13]

So let's reiterate: weight loss is hard because accumulated fat is very energy rich. Let's say you consume about 1,500 calories per day, manage to drop just 100 calories (or 6% or so of) total calorie intake, and increase fat burning by 300 calories a day. The net loss is 400 calories of (mostly) fat—a bit less than one-tenth of a pound. In 10 days, one can thus expect about a pound of fat to disappear, and in a year perhaps around 30 pounds. It isn't easy, but it always works with a bit of persistence and common sense: one ice cream root beer float (900 calories) can set you back at least two days worth of exercise and modest dietary prudence.

WATCH YOUR MOUTH, YOUNG MAN (AND WOMAN)

This book has largely focused on standard *medical* treatments for disease, but there is one part of the anatomy we have largely ignored that warrants at least brief attention: the mouth.

About 15 years ago, dentists began to suspect that their patients with bad oral health—usually inflammation of the gums (gingivitis) or the structures immediately around each of our teeth (bone, ligaments that attach the teeth to bone, and some specialized gum tissue)—also had a higher chance of getting heart attacks and even strokes. As time has gone by, epidemiologists and statisticians have studied the association. It is not only quite real, there is even a plausible set of mechanisms by which bacterial disease and inflammation in the mouth can accelerate atherosclerosis in multiple blood vessels in the body, especially in the heart and in the carotid arteries carrying blood to the brain.

A number of very good studies reveal this remarkable association—well thought out, carefully adjusted for other factors that might contribute to heart disease *and* bad oral health (e.g., smoking, age, and diet). The result of these studies is straightforward: the more tooth loss one has, the greater the quantity of bacteria in pockets buried deep in the gums around the roots of the teeth. Even the amount of effort put into maintaining oral health by a given individual is strongly associated with an increased risk of heart attack (and probably stroke), perhaps increasing the risk by 20% or more.[14] Because coronary disease and stroke are so common to start off with, this additional risk is hugely significant from the perspective of the individual and from the costs to the health care system at large.

Even in relatively young women of about age 50—who are at low risk for heart attack and stroke—there are clear links between the earliest lesions of atherosclerosis (not big enough to cause the compromise of blood flow but clearly the first few acts in the long drama of coronary and carotid disease) and poor dental hygiene.[15] In the women studied, the delicate lining of the carotid arteries can been seen by means of ultrasound imaging, and the more periodontal disease (measured very carefully by the number of pockets of bacteria around the teeth as found on physical examination or by X-rays), the thicker the carotid lining is—the very first measurable sign of atherosclerosis. This same thickening of the lining (called "intimal thickening") is correlated with a virtually identical process in the coronary arteries. In fact in studies done to date, periodontal disease was about as strong a determinant for carotid damage as was age. Put another way, periodontal disease dramatically accelerates the "aging" of blood vessels around the body.

How might this come about? The full story is far from in, but there are at least several probable mechanisms. First, chronic inflammation of any kind anywhere in the body seems to lead to inflammation of blood vessels everywhere in the body (acute or temporary inflammation does not). Since many people go years between visits to the dental hygienist or don't brush or floss regularly, the level of generalized inflammation in the mouth can be extremely high, stimulating the immune system in potent ways, which in turn causes the immune system to damage other portions of the body—much like the "autoimmune" diseases already discussed.

Next, the organisms that are found in the mouths of people with bad periodontal disease are also found in the atherosclerotic plaque in blood vessels of the heart and elsewhere.[16] It has been shown that these organisms gain access to the bloodstream from the mouth. How they end up specifically in atherosclerotic lesions is unclear, but it is easy to see that if the immune system is attacking them in the mouth, the same thing can occur in the arteries, and there is often substantial collateral damage when the white cells of the immune system and their powerful bacteria-destroying chemicals are on the march.

Third, as people with periodontitis start to lose teeth or have pain, they tend to change their diets. Fruits and vegetables—which require a lot of chewing before swallowing—are replaced by softer items that don't: eggs, fatty meats, candy, soft drinks. Thus, detrimental food choices may be made simply to avoid having to chew or put up with the discomfort of chewing.

Thus, the hypothesis that periodontal disease and vascular damage around the body (primarily via atherosclerosis) are related seems proven. What remains to be shown is whether actually *doing* something about the periodontal disease—flossing, brushing, and regular cleanings of plaque and tartar deep along the roots of the teeth— actually makes a difference in the incidence of coronary disease and stroke. A series of such studies is now under way. But, since there is no risk and very little cost to brushing and flossing (and even professional dental cleanings can be had for $100 or so), we believe it is prudent to do so as part of primary prevention. One thing is certain: you'll hold onto your teeth a lot longer, avoiding much pain and discomfort down the line.

EXAMINING THE PHYSICAL EXAM

For those of us in our fifties and sixties, when we were growing up the notion of an annual physical exam became the norm. We were advised, cajoled, or otherwise convinced that a yearly trip to the doctor "just to check things out" was a good idea, one that was strongly supported by the American Medical Association and your favorite family doctor. But, as with so many other things in medicine, the value of annual physical examination was never put to a controlled test until about 10 years ago. What we have learned is that, absent the established presence of one or more chronic diseases—that is, if you don't have high blood pressure, diabetes, excess weight (by far the three most common harmful conditions of modern society)—there may be *harm* to doing an annual physical exam.

Just how much harm a physical exam may do depends a bit on what constitutes that annual physical. Many people believe that a physical examination should consist of much more than just the doctor taking a careful history, listening to the heart and lungs, examining the joints, examining the skin for evidence of early skin cancers; some feel it should include things like annual electrocardiograms, chest X-rays, or perhaps annual stress tests.

These latter tests are clearly worse than worthless absent either an ongoing problem or patient complaints of new symptoms—for example, chest pain with exercise or, say, climbing a flight of stairs.

Despite the total absence of any data to support the use of diagnostic tests in the annual physical, many hospitals—some of them quite prestigious—recognize that such testing can be quite lucrative. And the so-called "complete physical" taken to its extreme—what is sometimes called an "executive physical"—is a lucrative source of income for those medical institutions. You can still get one at the Mayo Clinic for a few thousand dollars out of your own pocket (or, if you are in important executive, your company may be foolish enough to pay for it).

Let's look at an unfortunately common way the executive physical can go awry and do more harm than good. Suppose that at the age of 55 you decide that you're not satisfied with having a physical examination every three years—roughly the time interval between exams recommended by the U.S. Public Health Services' Preventive task force. So you decide to have a physical done every year and in the course of that physical you demand an exercise stress test "to be sure" everything is okay with your heart. You get on a treadmill, you exercise up to your maximal exercise capacity, and the physician measures not merely your heart rate but actually the change in the form of the electrical pulses in the heart.

Let's further say that during your treadmill some unusual wave patterns are seen on the continuous electrocardiogram recording being taken. There is no question that these abnormalities are often associated with a lack of adequate blood flow to the heart, including in patients with "angina" (exercise-related chest pain of a particular location and duration) and in people having actual "heart attacks" (damage to heart muscle due to lack of blood flow and other metabolic derangements that supervene during a heart attack).

But how often do "abnormal stress test" results occur in people *without* coronary disease or related heart troubles? The answer is much more than we used to think, perhaps in 5% to 15% of the population (depending on age and sex). Do these results imply a problem that needs to be further investigated or treated? The answer is definitively no.

Things get out of sensible control very quickly: it's almost always the case that the physician performing the stress test will recommend an invasive cardiovascular test if the stress test is "abnormal," even if the abnormality is just an incidental finding that is nothing more than an imperfection in the stress test itself (i.e., the test occasionally picks up strange electrical patterns that do not portend disease.)

If the patient is afraid (or foolish) enough to undergo a cardiac catherization, perhaps a few minor deposits of atherosclerosis in the coronary arteries are found. Now what? For many individuals—and not a few cardiologists who ought to know better—just as when we see calcium deposits in the pipes of our houses, we want to clean them out, and the physician wants to get rid of those fatty deposits or atherosclerotic deposits as well.

Perhaps the cardiologist will pass a catheter into the artery and remove or crush a small arterial plaque. In so doing, what we've now learned is that it makes the coronary arteries look much better during coronary catheterization and shortens the life span of the individual. We're not sure why, but it appears that in "cleaning the pipes," there is substantial risk of doing damage to the lining of the arteries. This actually leads to accelerated atherosclerosis a few months to a year or two down the line, which you don't recognize until you have a heart attack.

There is precious little evidence that routine screening physical examinations do any good, and indeed there is positive evidence for having only a few screening tests as we age (in the absence of symptoms).

A POCKET SUMMARY

In the United States and in most Western societies, the diseases and discomforts we face are mostly—though not exclusively—of our own doing. The preventive measures that make sense are limited:

- Dietary prudence (perhaps most important, what we *add* to our diets rather than what we take away).

- Modest routine exercise designed to maintain muscle tone and enhance cardiovascular fitness (and perhaps chasing away depression and improving overall sense of well-being).

- A very limited number of screening tests have been *proven*—as opposed to merely asserted—to be of benefit and with very low risk. The few screening tests that are actually beneficial are small in number: mammograms, bone density tests, and Pap smears for women, blood pressure and cholesterol measurements for everyone over the age of 45 or 50, colon cancer screening at long intervals (5 to 10 years or more), combined with yearly influenza vaccination, give the largest return in both absolute and relative terms compared to every other offering on the medical technology menu.

New screening technologies, based on advanced radiographic and even gene-profiling techniques, have yet to show any value. This is not to say that research and carefully controlled trials will not surprise us with new beneficial, life-saving preventive measures. But approach any new offering skeptically; be wary if the doctor can't answer the question, "What is the evidence that this new test will increase the quality or quantity of my life?"—or, worse, if he or she takes umbrage at your temerity for asking in the first place. Should either be the case find another doctor.

NOTES

1. This is true for tuna even though it has rather high levels of cholesterol. Oils from tuna flesh have protective factors in the form of long-chain fatty acids that counter the negative effects of cholesterol.
2. Atherosclerosis—literally "hardening of the arteries"—is now known to be, at best, an incomplete description of the disease processes involved in vascular damage, most of it irreversible. Even as recently as the mid-1990s there was little appreciation for the role that the immune system played in damaging blood vessels, because atherosclerosis was thought to be primarily related to cholesterol deposits and local blood vessel cell reaction to it. Instead, we now know that the white cells

that circulate in the blood for purposes of protecting us against infection can participate in and worsen the damage done by cholesterol deposits. Obviously, much more remains to be understood, but it is clear that atherosclerosis is much more than just clogging up the pipes with fat and cholesterol.

3. We really don't feel that you have to spend a premium on so-called organic fish oils, in part because the definitions of "organic oil" are spectacularly vague and spottily enforced at best.

4. D. Mozaffarian, E. B. Rimm, "Fish intake, contaminants, and human health: Evaluating the risks and the benefits," *Journal of the American Medical Association,* October 18, 2006; 296(15): 1885–1899.

5. H. E. Bays, "Safety considerations with omega-3 fatty acid therapy," *American Journal of Cardiology,* March 19, 2007; 99(6A): 35C–43C.

6. J. Montonen, R. Järvinen, P. Knekt, M. Heliövaara, A. Reunanen, National Public Health Institute, Helsinki FIN, Finland. "Consumption of sweetened beverages and intakes of fructose and glucose predict type 2 diabetes occurrence," *Journal of Nutrition,* June 2007; 137(6): 1447–1454. We include the abstract in this footnote, because the results have very important implications for millions of people who routinely consume soft drinks and similar foods or liquids.
The role of intakes of different sugars in the development of type 2 diabetes was studied in a cohort of 4,304 men and women aged 40–60 years and initially free of diabetes at baseline in 1967–1972. Food consumption data were collected using a dietary history interview covering the habitual diet during the previous year. The intakes of different sugars were calculated and divided in quartiles. During a 12-year follow-up, 177 incidents of type 2 diabetes cases were identified from a nationwide register. Combined intake of fructose and glucose was associated with the risk of type 2 diabetes but no significant association was observed for intakes of sucrose, lactose, or maltose. The relative risk between the highest and lowest quartiles of combined fructose and glucose intake was 1.87 (95% [CI] = 1.19, 2.93; P = 0.003). The corresponding relative risks between the extreme quartiles of consumption of food items contributing to sugar intakes were 1.69 (95% [CI] = 1.17, 2.43; P < 0.001) for sweetened berry juice and 1.67 (95% [CI] = 0.98, 2.87; P = 0.01) for soft drinks. Our findings support the view that higher intake of fructose and glucose and sweetened beverages may increase type 2 diabetes risk.

7. A. M. Hill, J. D. Buckley, K. J. Murphy, and P. R. C. Howe, "Combining fish-oil supplements with regular aerobic exercise improves body composition and cardiovascular disease risk factors," *American Journal of Clinical Nutrition,* May 2007; 85(5):1267–1274.

8. Males typically have more muscle mass as a percentage of total body weight than do females, and because muscle is the densest of all tissue (meaning it weighs more per cubic inch than any other tissue), the BMI for males of a given height is "normally" higher than the BMI for females.

9. Obviously some highly trained athletes with low body fat but lots of muscle can have BMIs that appear to be in the dangerous range but are not. Since such individuals are rather uncommon, we'll not discuss them further in this chapter.

10. L. Larun, L. V, Nordheim, E. Ekeland, K. B. Hagen, and F. Heian, "Exercise in prevention and treatment of anxiety and depression among children and young people," *Cochrane Database of Systematic Reviews: Reviews,* Issue 3 (Chichester, UK: John Wiley & Sons, Ltd., 2006).

11. M. Edmonds, H. McGuire, and J. Price, "Exercise therapy for chronic fatigue

syndrome," *Cochrane Database of Systematic Reviews: Reviews*, Issue 3 (Chichester, UK: John Wiley & Sons, Ltd., 2004).

12. L. Brosseau, L. MacLeay, V. A. Robinson, P. Tugwell, and G. Wells, "Intensity of exercise for the treatment of osteoarthritis," *Cochrane Database of Systematic Reviews: Reviews*, Issue 3 (Chichester, UK: John Wiley & Sons, Ltd., 2003).

13. Surely if a little exercise is good for you, more should be better, right? Not really. Think about the effect of excessive exercise, or exercise beyond this amount, and the incidents of damage to the joints. A lot of the data still remains somewhat speculative, despite the fact that many dozens if not many hundreds of studies have been done over the past 25 years. It clearly appears to be the case that the joints of the human body, particularly the knee, were not really designed for long-distance running beyond the age of about 40. This is especially true in people who are overweight. The best that can be said is that jogging activities neither help nor hurt the joints in people who are modestly overweight, but if you attempt to engage in long-distance running as an attempt to lose weight you likely will do damage to your knee joints. We simply don't have enough data to say whether anything beyond walking is truly damaging to the joints. But the evidence seems to be accumulating in that direction.

14. A. A. Bahekar, S. Singh, S. Saha, J. Molnar, and R. Arora, "The prevalence and incidence of coronary heart disease is significantly increased in periodontitis: A meta-analysis," *American Heart Journal*, November 2007; 154(5): 830–837.

15. B. Söder and M. Yakob, "Risk for the development of atherosclerosis in women with a high level of dental plaque and severe gingival inflammation," *International Journal of Dental Hygiene*, August 5, 2007; 5(3): 133–138.

16. H. A. Schenkein, S. E. Barbour, C. R. Berry, et al., "Invasion of human vascular endothelial cells by Actinobacillus actinomycetemcomitans via the receptor for platelet-activating factor," *Infectious Immunology*, 2000; 68: 5416–5419.

CHAPTER 11

How to Do More Good Than Harm

TO UNDERSTAND HOW RAPIDLY the practice of medicine has changed—and how we may have ended up doing more harm than good—consider this simple thought experiment. Imagine a time about three or four decades ago, back when the kind Dr. Welby was the TV icon of the family physician. Many of today's middle-aged physicians were about to enter medical school and then grapple with changes that would completely skew the health care landscape

Infectious disease of all types was thought to be near extinction. New antibiotics for curing serious bacterial infections were being released at the rate of several a year with hundreds of candidate drugs in the pipeline. Only a few antibiotics were actually necessary to treat the vast majority of infections because bacterial resistance to drugs had only begun to emerge as a serious problem. Tuberculosis was a disease in decline with the prospect of its ultimate eradication as well; public health departments were correctly given credit for this significant advance and it was anticipated that epidemiologists and public health nurses would play an important role in the final elimination of most infectious disease scourges.

There were about a dozen medications to treat hypertension, by then already realized as a major cause of heart disease and stroke, both exploding in prevalence. Most doctors were familiar with most of these drugs and rarely needed to consult a cardiologist or hypertension specialist.

The 1964 Surgeon General's report, written by Luther Terry, on the dangers of cigarette smoking were finally starting to have an impact on behaviors, and a few hearty souls went out "jogging" because some studies picked up by the popular press seemed to show that exercise decreased the chances that one would develop coronary disease. It seemed that infectious disease was disappearing and that the greatest threats to health in the rich world were diseases of self-abuse: eating too much, not exercising enough, and using dangerous recreational drugs—all of which were seen as avoidable or remediable.

Imaging techniques were pretty much limited to variations on the plain old X-ray; a primitive form of tomography (the "T" in CAT scan) enabled radiologists to see lesions in the lungs, bone and sometimes brain that were 2 centimeters (an inch or so) in diameter, but pictures of the soft tissues in the abdomen were impossible to obtain. A few cardiologists (there weren't very many back then; internists filled that role) were experimenting with a technique called catheterization where a thin plastic tube was carefully threaded into the aorta and, with a little luck, into the much tinier coronary arteries themselves. Dye could be injected into the ventricle of the heart so that the function of large structures such as valves could be visualized and simultaneously the cardiac bypass machine was perfected so that surgeons could stop the heart to repair or replace damaged heart valves and—tepidly at first—even blockages in some of the coronary arterial tree. A few radiologists were visualizing blockages in the arteries carrying blood to the legs or intestinal tract using very much the same techniques, but they were largely considered experimental.

Morbidity—loosely speaking "damage or suffering" from these procedures—was common, and mortality was hardly unheard of. For the most part, little could be done for patients with severe coronary disease, and when they had a heart attack, the patient was put to bed and given aspirin while everyone hoped for the best but expected the worst. Dr. Christian Barnard tried to perform a heart transplant in 1967 on a dentist, Louis Washkansky, who suffered from diabetes and the effects of multiple heart attacks. A team of more than two dozen people worked for 10 hours, giving the good dentist another 18 days of life before his transplanted heart was rejected by his own body's immune system, a problem that proved stubbornly resistant to treatment.

The "war on cancer" was starting up and cures were seen as all but inevitable with new drugs that were being found by empirical testing, first in animals and then in humans. No one thought much of testing people for cancer before they were obviously symptomatic with the disease. No one could have anticipated how difficult achieving a "cure" in most patients with metastatic cancer would be.

In psychiatry, psychoanalysis—long, expensive, and variably effective for anxiety, depression, and schizophrenia—was falling out of favor as new classes of drugs for these all-too-common mental illnesses started coming onto the market. By 1980, state "mental" hospitals started to close, as the vast majority of patients—even those with the worst psychotic disease, patients literally out of touch with reality— could be treated as outpatients with medications like thorazine. Indeed, the treatment of psychotic disorders was arguably one of the greatest breakthroughs at the time. Before the late 1970s little could be done for such patients but warehousing in asylums.

From a systematic standpoint, delivery of health care was patchy, but most working people could afford an office visit or a short hospitalization especially because employer-provided health insurance—an outgrowth of generous tax breaks legislated by Congress—was more or less universal among people with full-time jobs. Care for indigents was often provided by public health clinics. Almost everyone was satisfied with their health care and saw a future of increasing disease-free longevity for most. Medical care was a very private affair based on a close relationship between the patient and their family physician who often had also cared for their parents and was providing most of the medical care for their children; there were no television or newspaper advertisements hawking the latest allergy, blood pressure, or erectile dysfunction drugs.

And it was all done at a cost of a few hundred billion dollars a year—perhaps 5 or 6% of the Gross Domestic Product of the time.

As this book goes to market the world of medicine appears to have turned upside down. Today, virtually everyone with coronary disease can expect to have their blockages bypassed or crushed with a sophisticated angioplasty catheter, and if multiple heart attacks have reduced the heart muscle to a quivering floppy bag that can't pump, heart transplants are available almost routinely now that our ability to manage rejection has been made almost as simple as taking antibiotics.

The rate of progress in the treatment of serious psychiatric disease seems to have come to a halt, not because we haven't discovered new drugs nor failed in more carefully tailoring drug choices but because we've learned that psychotic disease—schizophrenia in particular—is actually a progressive, degenerative brain disease. As with Parkinson's disease, we can control symptoms for a good long while, but ultimately the patient succumbs to the disease, often becoming mute and motionless: the "catatonic state."

But infectious diseases have boomed, both in number of new organisms and number of people dying from them. Many of the organisms causing bacterial infections that were susceptible to one of a handful of antibiotics are now resistant to just about every one of the many dozens of antibiotics on the market (including new classes of antibiotics that work in novel ways compared to more-or-less similar drugs of the 1970s and early 1980s), and tuberculosis is not only much more common now than in 1970 but is often much more difficult to treat as that organism too has acquired the ability to resist treatment. One form of tuberculosis—called "extensively drug resistant tuberculosis" (XDR-TB)—may prove to be fatal in almost everyone who has it. The first few hundred cases started to be recognized only within the past year or two. Food-borne infections are, if anything, more diverse and probably more common than ever, perhaps because of the way we raise animals in enormous feedlots (up to 50,000 head of cattle are no longer unusual in an area less than a square mile) or chicken houses (where birds are given half of a square foot each from birth to slaughter a few weeks later).

Besides HIV/AIDS that suddenly appeared in the early 1980s, we now have discovered a plethora of new infectious diseases such Ebola, Marburg, cryptosporidiosis, SARS, hantavirus and hemorrhagic E. Coli, all of them frequently fatal. There are dozens of newly appreciated (though doubtless ancient) viruses that most physicians can't even pronounce whose significance is still not understood. A novel type of influenza called H5N1 was recognized in birds in the late 1990s and has been fatal to hundreds of millions of them, but it has also killed nearly two hundred humans, including young healthy people who normally shake off the "flu."

Because we lack even a rudimentary real-time disease monitoring system in the United States, we don't know *when* infectious disease is spreading or when a small outbreak—that *could* turn into a large epidemic if not detected early—occurs until many days or even weeks after the initial event. Much to everyone's surprise, the very successes of public health and vaccine-preventable disease strategies in the 1950s through the early 1970s lead to a de-funding of public health offices around the country. To the extent that the United States had the capacity to identify and counter disease outbreaks, it began to quickly atrophy.

The accompanying lack of situational awareness—the bedrock of prevention—can lead us to both overreact and underreact. For example, in the case of the new strain of influenza, starting about two years ago many "experts" predicted dire consequences from a worldwide pandemic not dissimilar to what happened in 1918 when a new strain of influenza killed more than 5% of world human population (and an unknown number of animals and birds). At the same time, others counseled caution, recognizing that the new avian flu shared a common surface constituent with one of the human strains of flu that has been circulating for decades, meaning that it is likely that the vast majority of humans are already immune to the new flu because of previous exposure to its near cousin or because the commonly used yearly influenza vaccine probably provides protection against H5N1. It appears to be the case that worldwide literally hundreds of millions of people have been *infected* by H5N1 but almost none have become ill because the individuals' immune systems eliminate the virus before it can cause much damage.[1] Yet, in the U.S. alone, billions of dollars have been spent on stockpiling medication—of questionable efficacy—against H5N1 and on developing a new vaccine which is likely years away from introduction for human use. A simple electronic reporting system enabling doctors to look for and report rare cases of unusually severe manifestations of "flu-like illness" would probably define the actual threat of H5N1 to humans with high confidence, yet federal and state public health officials are reluctant—even resistant—to implement one.[2]

And cancer is more common than ever, and average mortality rates have scarcely budged in patients who have metastatic disease. Save for those people whose disease has been identified by screening, it's hard to point to many therapeutic successes with cancer—and in some cancer types we may be harming more people than we are helping.

Disparities in health care delivery have never been worse; at any given time at least 15% of Americans will have no health insurance, and many others simply skip buying it because it is so expensive. For those who do have access to health care, the chances of being on the receiving end of an invasive procedure for heart disease, degenerative arthritis, prostate cancer, and at least a half-dozen other common problems among the Medicare population—that group which is universally insured—varies by about a factor of 10 from place to place across town or across the country, yet there is no difference in overall outcomes from these diseases. Nearly four decades of data that prove this striking point go largely ignored.

Far fewer Americans are satisfied with their health care and are stymied by paperwork, referral forms, ever-changing health plans and physicians, and a blizzard of direct-to-patient advertising of countless drugs on television.

And it's all being done at a cost of a few trillion dollars a year— somewhere between 16 and 18% of the entire GDP of the United States without much change in longevity or quality of health. Health care inflation—briefly contained in the 1980s when HMOs first came onto the scene—is now fully two or three times the rate of inflation for other services and goods in the U.S. economy.

Just about all of our expectations about life-threatening disease has changed completely; health care is probably the largest "industry" in the U.S., and will consume 1 out of every 5 dollars expended within the next 10 years unless something changes. As the population ages—the demographic shift toward an older population is all but inevitable—costs will increase unless we are smarter about the way we make medical treatment decisions toward the end of life. Spending even more money is not the solution; and it probably isn't in the cards in any case as employers are cutting back the coverage they offer their staffs. It is increasingly the case that when people change jobs they may or may not have the same (or any) health insurance coverage. Health insurance coverage has become so expensive that many people hold on to jobs they don't like, or decline opportunities where their skills might be better utilized, for fear of losing this precious employment benefit.

TURNING THINGS AROUND: THE PAYERS AND PLAYERS

There will be no easy solutions to make medicine in the U.S. cost-effective, or to guarantee a process that will rein in inherently unknowable health care costs as disease patterns change and new technologies are discovered, many of them serendipitously, with high up-front costs. However, we believe that the detailed studies published in the medical literature that have been reviewed in this book provide a series of guidelines or requirements for the "next generation" of health care delivery in the United States. Were we to all start with a clean slate (and of course we can't) most of us would envision a healthcare delivery system that:

- Provides medical care—including diagnostics, invasive procedures, therapies, medications and preventive services—based on clear scientific evidence.

- Removes the existing, indefensible variability especially in expensive and often unproven procedures.

- Stresses prevention over treatment and rewards both patients and physicians for avoiding illness.

- Provides health care insurance coverage for virtually everyone.

- Takes advantage of modern, secure communication through the Internet to make every patient's medical records and history available to authorized users.

- Incorporates research not as an academic process but as a process inherent in daily medical practice so that practical improvements in efficiency and patient satisfaction can be achieved based on the needs of specific patient populations.

- One that eliminates the overhead costs associated with hundreds of different health-care systems, insurers and payers.

It sounds hard, doesn't it? But, there is an example of a real-world, quasi-independent health care system that meets most of these requirements: the Veterans Administration (VA) and its archipelago of hospitals and clinics. Problems abound at the VA, but they are almost exclusively administrative, having to do with eligibility requirements and the like. But on the other hand, the VA has been transformed in the past few decades, partially as a result of affiliation with local university medical schools, a robust research program funded within the Veterans Administration itself, and by attracting top-flight physicians who are paid not by how much they do but based on the appropriateness of their care. The VA hasn't the money or resources to waste on unnecessary procedures; and headlines to the contrary aside, the day-to-day delivery of health care meets the needs of hundreds of thousands of veterans who often have very complex, interacting medical problems.

Among the advances in medicine led by the VA that even the best health-maintenance organizations such as Kaiser-Permanente are struggling to establish are:

- Electronic medical records, available to authorized users (physicians, nurses, and some administrators) on a 24/7 basis over the Internet.

- Digitized X-rays, electrocardiograms, CAT scans and MRI scans, laboratory reports and medication lists, also accessible from just about every VA clinic and at the homes of health care providers who may get called about a patient at night.

- Internal reviews of new technologies and procedures as they come online to identify patients who will benefit and patients who may be harmed.

- Purchasing medications in large quantities from pharmaceutical companies, thus obtaining best prices. This is especially important as in recent years money spent on medication has increased in both absolute and relative terms: a greater percentage of an ever larger health care budget is now devoted to pharmaceuticals than ever before.

And, among the accomplishments of the VA, truly groundbreaking research (often done with associated university hospitals) that guided application of new technologies in the rest of medicine are:

- Coronary artery bypass, including very clear criteria for who benefits from the operation and who does better with medication (or in fact does worse with bypass)

- Optimizing treatment of hypertension and high cholesterol

- Preventing medical errors such as "wrong-side" operations, incorrect dosing of potentially dangerous medications and other avoidable errors that result in more than 100,000 deaths per year in community, academic and specialty hospitals outside of the VA system

- Training practicing physicians to fulfill administrative roles while maintaining their clinical duties, thus cutting costs and introducing rational policies into daily health care delivery

- Implementing a practical "outcomes research" program for virtually all medical and psychiatric services at the VA

It is important to point out that the VA deals with a specialized population that is overwhelming male and mostly elderly, and thus its profoundly successful experiences may not apply to other health care systems. But, given the complexity and severity of illness of patients within its system of hospitals, the VA has shown what can be accomplished with science-based medicine.

Taking a closer look at the requirements for the next-generation of health care in the U.S., we can identify what has been done, what needs to be done, and where the roadblocks are. We'll then cover some specific recommendations on how to fix the biggest holes in medical care delivery.

REVAMPING MEDICAL EDUCATION: UNDERGRADUATE AND POST-GRADUATE STUDIES

Medical schools and post-graduate residency training programs stress the importance of "evidence based medicine" (EBM) in their course requirements (begging the obvious question: what kind of kind of scientific knowledge was imparted to the nation's young doctors before "evidence" was used?). For example, the University of Pittsburgh—which touts its stature by noting that it is seventh among all educational institutions in total funding received for research from the National Institutes of Health (likely as much based on politics as on merit)—writes in its 2006–2007 "Fact Book" for incoming students[3]:

> An important skill set for physicians today is being able to interpret and evaluate new findings reported in the medical literature and to apply these advances to real-life circumstances. For instance, the ability to understand and rapidly evaluate conflicting reports on a new or even a commonly used drug is increasingly important in daily patient care.
>
> Evidence-based medicine—an ongoing focus of our curriculum—teaches students how to critically evaluate the medical literature and to

use medical databases to make patient care decisions based on best-known practice.

What kind of substance—that is, actual course work requirements—is behind the rhetoric? The answer is not easy to find, but the data strongly suggests that few medical schools are very serious when it comes to providing their students with the fundamental tools necessary to continue their understanding of EBM in articles. The point is not a trivial one because rote information—based on experience or studies up to any given point in time—probably has a useful half-life of 5 years or less, as new data, technologies and treatments accumulate rapidly in medicine. The Mayo Clinic Journal notes that:

"EBM has appropriately focused attention on critical appraisal of clinical research. A result of this movement is that medical specialists must improve their grasp of epidemiological and statistical principles. Despite this motivation, statistical knowledge has remained poor among clinicians."[4]

Thus, one way to see if medical schools "walk the walk" instead of merely "talking the talk" is to ask: how many schools require some number of hours of training in biostatistics or epidemiology. The answer is hard to come by as there is no uniform survey of all medical schools (partially because medical schools cover certain core items under different course names). The most authoritative source—and one which readers can query online—is American Association of Medical Colleges "curriculum directory."[5] One way to see if medical schools truly believe that some knowledge of statistical biostatistics—the key basis for physician understanding of the flood of data published in new scientific studies and its applicability to individual patients—is to query the AAMC database and compare offerings in "biostatistics or epidemiology" with the more traditional course requirements in anatomy and physiology. The results are not encouraging.

Of 125 U.S. medical schools, all *claim* to teach biostatistics as part of other courses.[6]

But digging just a bit deeper into the AAMC database, biostatistics doesn't fair very well as Figure 11-1 shows.

FIGURE 11-1. AAMC course listings with hours required.

Course	Total Number of Schools Reporting Some Required Hours	Percent of 125 US Medical Schools Reporting
Anatomy	66	53%
Biochemistry	51	41%
Biostatistics	23	18%
Cell Biology/Histology	74	59%
Genetics	43	34%
Immunology/Micro	47	38%
Neuroanatomy	73	58%
Pathology	31	25%
Pharmacology	26	21%
Physiology	57	46%

While reporting is not required and hence firm conclusions may be difficult to draw, biostatistics apparently fairs the worst among "core" courses. Most medical schools still require rote memorization of anatomy and cell biology (and the overwhelming majority of practicing physicians will tell you that they remember little of the anatomy they were forced to memorize, save for that which applies to their area of specialty); only 18% require course work in biostatistics. The University of Pittsburgh doesn't require a course of biostatistics despite its flowery rhetoric, and it is far from alone even among leading medical schools.

These numbers are consistent with a recent study on post-graduate (residents') knowledge of statistical concepts, which in turn reflects on practicing physicians' ability to properly interpret new medical literature. Two hundred seventy-seven residents in 11 different programs were asked to answer 20 questions about statistical information found in articles (and not a single actual calculation was required, so there was no need for the residents to have any knowledge of *how* to do statistical analysis, but rather to correctly answer questions about the *meaning* of statistical conclusions in published papers). On average, they answered only 8 out of 20 questions correctly.[7] But the news is even worse: few residents (about 10% of those surveyed) could correctly interpret the most important statistical results that differentiated the usefulness of various treatments for a specific illness.

Put another way, the vast majority of residents don't know how to read a medical paper. It is little wonder that physicians misuse new information that they haven't already been forced to memorize or otherwise regurgitate. Thinking through new evidence simply isn't part of medical training in general. It's long past time that hours wasted in memorizing obscure anatomical structures (soon forgotten and of little relevance except in certain specialties, e.g., neurosurgery, where the information can be taught as part of post-graduate training) be replaced with a statistics requirement for all students. If your doctor doesn't know how to apply new information in the course of his or her career, given the accelerating pace of new technological offerings, the chances of more harmful than good medical care being delivered only increases.

PROVIDING MEDICAL CARE BASED ON SCIENTIFIC EVIDENCE

It is not enough to have "evidence based medicine" but also "medicine based on evidence," that is, knowledge that is obtained in realistic practice situations recognizing that one size does not fit all. Indeed, this is a frequent complaint of many physicians: "what's published in the medical journals doesn't apply to my practice."

And sometimes, they are right. Since practices and the patients within those practices vary, a study done at an academic medical center may or may not apply to a high-end practice on the Upper East Side of New York City or to a homeless clinic in Chelsea. Thus, it will be necessary for data to be gathered from a variety of practices, analyzed and provided to physicians based on the demographics of their populations. We'll illustrate in Figure 12-2 how that might be done.

But let's start with the clearest example of science-based medicine: prevention. We know that screening for a small set of diseases and some counseling (for example, to encourage exercise) is cost-effective. The recommendations for screening for breast cancer, high blood pressure and cholesterol apply across just about every demographic group of adults—rich, poor, black, white, Hispanic—that one can name. What is surprising is how long it has taken to find even the very limited number—about 10—of screening and prevention techniques that have stood the test of prospective, controlled studies and are recommended by national-level health officials in multiple countries. We summarize the screening tests and other preventive measures for adults that have been proven to be cost-effective after years of painstaking analysis in Figure 11-2.

The Public Health Service, in collaboration with a similar group in Canada has made recommendations *and* warnings of what *not* to do (see Figure 11-2).[8]

FIGURE 11-2. Public Health Service recommendations and warnings.

Screening Tests/Exams

1. *Hypertension:* screen blood pressure periodically.
2. *Obesity:* screen height and weight periodically.
3. *Lipids:* Total cholesterol and HDL—Men 35–70 years and women 45–70 years—every 5 years.
4. *Breast Cancer:* Mammogram age 40–70—every 1–2 years.
5. *Cervical Cancer:* Pap Smear every 1–3 years after 3 normal Paps within 5 years (unless S/P non-cancer hysterectomy). First Pap 3 years after first intercourse or age 21. May discontinue after 65 if persistently normal.
6. *Colon cancer screen:* Age 50 + . Fecal occult blood testing yearly or sigmoidoscopy (or colonoscopy) every 5–10 years.
7. *Chlamydia Infection Screening:* Routinely for all sexually active women age 25 or younger and other asymptomatic women at increased risk.
8. *Osteoporosis Screening:* Bone density testing one time in women age 65 + and age 60–65 if at increased risk of osteoporotic fractures.
9. *Abdominal Aortic Aneurysm Screening:* One time ultrasonography

in men age 65–75 who have ever smoked. (Not recommended in men who have never smoked or in women.)

10. *Prostate Cancer Screening:* Insufficient evidence to recommend for or against screening by PSA or digital rectal exam.

Vaccinations

1. *Tetanus—diphtheria* (Td) booster: every 10 years. May substitute 1 dose Tetanus-diphtheria-pertussis (Tdap) age 18–65.
2. *Pneumococcal vaccine:* once at age 65 + .
3. *Influenza vaccine:* yearly at age 50 + .
4. *Mumps-Measles-Rubella (MMR):* 1–2 doses if born during or after 1957.
5. *Varicella:* 2 doses of non-immune or not previously infected.

Chemoprevention and Counseling

1. *Health Promotion Questionnaire*—yearly, with special attention to
   * Smoking and alcohol
   * Substance abuse
   * Depression
   * High risk behavior for HIV/STDs
   * Physical activity
   * Healthy diet (low fat)
   * MVA prevention—Seatbelt use, avoidance of alcohol/substances
   * Falls in elderly
   * Risk of unintended pregnancy
2. *Aspirin for the Primary Prevention of Cardiovascular Events:* Discuss with adults at increased risk of coronary heart disease (men age 40 + , post-menopausal women and younger with major risk factors). Discuss both risks and benefits.
3. *Screening Tests for At Risk Populations:*
   * HIV testing, screening for Syphilis (RPR), gonorrhea if high risk.

(continues)

FIGURE 11-2. (*continued*)

- Diabetes screening: Fasting blood sugar if high risk especially if hypertension or hyperlipidemia is present.
4. *Vision:* age 65 + by Snellen chart alone.
5. *Hearing:* age 65 + by questioning (and not requiring formal testing).

Equally surprising is the vast number of screening tests that have been tried and—just like many of the medical procedures and therapies we have covered in this book—that have been found to be worthless or perhaps even worse-than-worthless. The root of the problem is, once again, the lack of adequate data in real-world practice settings. A secondary problem is compliance: for some preventative measures such as mammography, the track record is good; for others—such as adult vaccinations for influenza and a few other highly communicable infectious diseases—it is miserable. And there are probably good reasons for this variability: physicians are poorly reimbursed for time spent in explaining preventive testing and then counseling patients based on the results. Another may be the motivation from fear. "Cancer" is a word that evokes an emotional reaction in everyone; "influenza" does not. Thus, it may be the case that women obtain mammograms (and, unfortunately, males permit their doctors to do PSA screening tests for prostate cancer) because they hope to avoid even having to think about cancer (and for mammography, we know that screening works well, almost to the point of eliminating death from the most common form of breast cancer if it is detected early enough).

Yet, if there ever is a serious epidemic of influenza—and we haven't enough knowledge to be able to predict these rare but catastrophic events—vaccination will be critical to prevent spread of the disease and also for one other important and oft-overlooked reason: it will help doctors know what a patient does not have if the patient has been vaccinated against the common circulating strains of viruses that also cause respiratory symptoms, fever, and muscle aches—or what is known as "influenza-like" illness.

There are several ways to increase compliance with vaccinations: first, individuals can have their insurance premiums reduced if they receive recommended vaccinations. Second, physicians and nurses should—as a matter of good medical practice and protection of patients—get vaccinated themselves, lest they become a vector for disease. Regrettably, only about 30% of physicians and nurses get yearly influenza shots. In our view, this is negligence in its purest form, as it means that the health care provider can acquire a highly communicable disease and then spread it to patients.

We know from the basic science that vaccination not only largely prevents acquiring a particular disease but that also if one does get ill despite having been vaccinated the illness is milder and the infected individual sheds far less virus so that others are not at risk from close contact (as might occur in the examination room). That a physician or nurse can have influenza yet be working in a hospital where, by definition, there are already hundreds of frail patients who could easily die if they acquire influenza on top of their other medical problems is unconscionable.

There are probably other screening tests and preventative measures still waiting to be discovered, and the clinic of tomorrow might be the "laboratory" where they are identified. Culling and analyzing the rich source of information in encounters between patients and their health care provider might be done in an automated fashion. We'll describe that as well; think of it as the realization of practical "medicine based evidence."

Of course, many physicians will resist sharing information about their practices. They may fear that they'll be identified as expensive "outliers" on the spectrum of costs for patient care, or may fear malpractice suits or even accusations of fraud by either doing "too much" or "too little," but we believe there is a way around this problem, largely based on the experience at the VA.

A second clear requirement of science-based medical practice is the elimination in the variation of use of oft-expensive procedures such as coronary stents or coronary artery bypass in patients with minimal heart disease, neck fusion for chronic pain but in the absence of threatened neurological damage. There can be no excuse for society to continue to pay for medical services of any kind that are either unproven or whose efficacy is unclear, or even worse when there are known life-threatening complications that must be balanced against an uncertain benefit. When new uses for established technologies are proposed or offered *or* new technologies are introduced, they should be reported as part of a clinical trial. There is much encouraging precedence for this approach. Most practicing oncologists—not just those in academic medical centers—have been doing so for more than 2 decades to evaluate new drugs and therapies, and there is no reason that the same can't be adopted by all medical specialties.

Because certain medical specialties subsume the lion's share of unproven technologies, they can be expected to undergo the greatest changes. There is little doubt that because lots of money is involved, change will be resisted, or as has been shown many times in the past, physicians may find a way to continue business-as-usual despite the absence of evidence for benefit in much of what they are doing. Much and perhaps most of the $2.5 trillion dollars spent annually finds its way into practitioners in the specialties of cardiology, diagnostic radiology, orthopedics and neurosurgery.

THE NEED FOR UNIVERSAL COVERAGE

While we should recognize that there will always be some people left out or who simply opt out of any comprehensive health insurance scheme, but it doesn't take much thinking—or much of a heart—to realize that a wealthy country such as the United States can do much better than having 15 to 20% of its population at any given time going without access to basic health care services, nor can we countenance a system that forces individuals to depend on emergency rooms when long-standing chronic medical conditions finally become intolerable. These end-stage complications are often near-impossible to treat, though that doesn't stop the expenditure of enormous quantities of money in the end-stages of various diseases in patients who get their last-ditch medical care in this way in emergency rooms and community hospitals. There is no way to force someone—especially someone who is poor—to pay for health care coverage. This will have to be provided by government either via incentives or subsidies of other types.

We believe this is not only affordable, it is essential. The most important reason for doing so isn't merely a matter of fairness, important as we all believe it to be, but rather because we all share in the benefits of universal coverage. There are many examples; let's consider a few. Chronic diseases such as diabetes may smolder for years before complications such as renal failure bring a patient near death. Although we don't have precise data, most health care analysts believe that the vast majority of these complications can be prevented, sparing much suffering and money in the long run. Forestalling the need for dialysis for even a few years by achieving reasonable control of blood sugar and the almost inevitable accompanying hypertension at a few hundred dollars a year would save tens of thousands of dollars. Prevention—or at least long delay—of heart disease, stroke, and atherosclerosis of the arteries in the lower limbs is demonstrably achievable and the cost savings are profound.

If communicable infectious disease continues its resurgence, failure to recognize it in the earliest phase of an outbreak will mean far more suffering, death across the population. A new communicable strain of influenza can appear across the country in a few weeks or less given the daily movements of hundreds of thousands of people by air travel and millions more by other means of conveyance. An early encounter with a health care provider who recognizes and reports an unusually severe respiratory disease can save many lives. We saw such an example when the source of previously unknown hantavirus pulmonary syndrome (HPS) came about when just one physician saw two young adult patients in the same town with sudden-onset of a fatal pneumonia (fortunately, because the patients were Native Americans they received free health care). By reporting these two cases, public health officials rapidly identified a half-dozen others that had gone unreported, leading to a quick investigation of possible sources of infection. While HPS couldn't be treated very well once someone was infected, it could easily be prevented by avoiding the source: a small field mouse ubiquitous in much of the United States. It is difficult to know how many lives were saved and panic avoided, but most infectious disease experts believe that the epidemic could have killed many dozens of people if they had no access to health care and instead died at home, written off as "unexplained community acquired pneumonia." And HPS turned out not to be communicable from person to person; had it been, the carnage would have been magnified many fold unless the new disease had been identified early in its course.

But savings also accrue via paths other than expenditures within the health care system. An almost certain benefit of universal coverage is maintaining an individual's productivity within society. Surely most of us would agree that a 60 year old diabetic who is working rather than spending 3 days a week getting dialysis is a benefit to us all.

Finally, unless we are willing to allow people with advanced disease to simply die when they develop life-threatening complications, more and more health care dollars will be spent with less and less return. No one would advocate such a policy in a compassionate society, and as we hope we've made clear, the problem isn't too little money to go around, its too much money being spent in the wrong places for the wrong interventions. So we offer one caveat to the otherwise compelling rationale for universal coverage: if we provide health care coverage to more people but continue to engage in costly, unproven or dangerous therapies we'll subject some large number of people to more harm, while driving up health care costs even further.

Letting a Thousand Laboratories Bloom

The overwhelming majority of physicians across all specialties learn and practice largely by rote. This is not to say that physicians are thoughtless, unintelligent automatons, but rather that few have the time or scientific backgrounds to analyze published data and create their own computer decision-models to help divine the best choice among many options. Truly fine clinicians—generally the ones doctors themselves choose to go to when they themselves get ill—actually perform the latter in their minds as a matter of innate talent, but they are few and far between. And, no one can discount the equally rare physician who is blessed with a near perfect memory and can recall practically everything they have ever read, all-the-while continuing to read vast quantities of papers in their fields.

But, because physicians have so many encounters with so many problems they record very valuable data in their medical records, almost always by writing—scrutable, as legend correctly has it, only to themselves. If one takes a step back, it isn't hard to realize that there is an immense lost opportunity here: gigabytes of data in every physician's office, almost none of it available for analysis and sharing.

Consider the following still-unanswered questions in medicine: do people who take anti-inflammatory drugs (aspirin, ibuprofen, etc.) on a chronic basis (say for arthritis or back pain) have a lower incidence of colon cancer? Of stroke? Of serious heart disease? Of Alzheimer's disease?

We could probably answer all of these questions definitively—right down to which age and racial groups, gender, and socio-economic and geographic strata do in fact benefit and those who do not— if we could just get an anonymous electronic record of those patients taking aspirin and following them along until their old age (or death). For all intents and purposes, a "natural experiment" is taking place in every clinic, large and small, across the country. Perhaps people who take aspirin every day to prevent heart disease also have a decreased propensity to other degenerative diseases or even for some kinds of cancer. On the other hand, perhaps they also suffer more cases of fatal gastrointestinal bleeding—a well-known side effect of even low-dose aspirin, especially in the elderly—that wipes out any additional benefit. We simply don't know.

But what we *do* know is that this precious data is being recorded in patient records. And, it is almost inaccessible to researchers if written on paper or lost entirely when a physician retires and fails to pass medical records on to someone else.

While we realize that most physicians lack the training—or desire!—to do research, we also believe that it's possible to mine data from individual practices. This can be done while protecting patient confidentiality and only the select information could be passed on to researchers who can analyze the information for answers to the questions posed above. In addition, such research will help identify unnecessary expenditures and care while providing continuous feedback to physicians that will help to improve their own efficiency. It is highly likely in our view that better outcomes will be the result.

ELECTRONIC MEDICAL RECORDS AND THE INTERNET

One of the holy grails of medicine has been the development of a robust, user-friendly electronic medical record (EMR) for the many "sub-communities" within medicine that have a "need to know" certain pieces of information. Physicians clearly need access to their notes, past medical history, recent examination findings, medication lists, allergies, laboratory blood test results (of which there are many dozen) and imaging studies such as chest X-rays, CAT scans, MRI scans and even pictures of microscopic biopsies. Nurses may need access to similar information, while insurance companies might want to know what kind of coverage is provided by a particular policy so that referrals to appropriate consultants and laboratories can be made.

By some estimates, 20% of all medical costs are generated by the repetition of unnecessary tests or the prescription of medications that have previously been unsuccessful. This figure doesn't include the inconvenience to the patient—time, stress, delay in diagnosis and treatment and their attendant frustration—and the side effects of unneeded or potentially risky procedures.

A more-or-less standardized EMR can be "queried" for a nearly limitless stream of valuable administrative and scientific information. As noted above, there remain important questions about very common conditions—stroke, cancer prevention of multiple types, degenerative problems and Alzheimer's disease—whose origins and treatments might be clarified by looking at correlations among age, medications, behaviors, diet, other medical conditions, and so forth. With an EMR—and of course, appropriate protections for patient confidentiality—scientific investigations along these lines could be automated, or at least made much easier.

The Mayo Clinic in Rochester was the first large, self-contained medical care system to employ a "unified" medical record—a large file for every patient. When conceived in the 1940s and 1950s, paper was the only recording medium available, but the thoughtful planners at Mayo recognized its benefit nonetheless. The record would literally follow every patient around the clinic via old pneumatic vacuum tubes, so that even if a patient had multiple appointments in the sprawling Mayo campus in one day, their chart would, quite literally, precede them to their next appointment. Efficient transfer of information from one specialist to another became daily practice more than five decades ago (though whether or not this led to more appropriate use of Mayo's always-cutting-edge medical technology is a separate question).

With the advent of the unified patient record, individual patient's files at Mayo were "coded" by professionals in the medical records department such that all patients with a given diagnosis—let's say some rare rheumatologic or autoimmune disease—could be retrieved (albeit with some effort of running through miles of shelves of paper) for research. Thus, the Mayo was able to address fundamental questions of epidemiology of disease—who gets it? How common is it (or its "incidence")? How long does it last (the "prevalence"?)—all while looking at how survival and quality of life were improved or perhaps made worse by various interventions, proving the principle that scientific research can take place in the context of daily medical care.

Today the same thing can be done electronically; but it gets even better. "Coding" or "classification" of patient charts by disease can be automated since almost all disease entities have an agreed "diagnosis code" assigned to them. Keywords can be found by computer (and refined by very clever algorithms) to accurately categorize patients by demographics, disease group or individual disease. The boon to scientific research from even small clinics or individual physicians' offices doing the same thing—without the need for large laboratories and grants—is obvious.

Reducing Payment Disparities Among Health Care Specialties

Few people outside of health care are aware of large differences in earnings among physicians. Most patients visiting their primary care physician assume he or she is doing quite well financially, and compared to average take-home pay your family doctor is rather well paid: around $160,000 a year in 2004[9] (although there is a wide variation in earnings; 15% of full time family doctors earn less than $100,000- per year). But the future survival of primary care medicine (PCM) is in doubt. Fewer than 8% of medical students chose a residency in family practice in 2005, down from 14% just 5 years earlier (by definition, almost all graduates of a family practice residency will practice primary care medicine as there is little in the way of sub-specialization within family practice, so it is a good indicator of physician workforce supply in PCM for the next few decades).

There are several reasons for the decline of interest in PCM among students, and leading among them is the substantially greater earning potential in non–primary care specialties combined with a median debt of approximately $140,000 upon completing medical school. Even though specialty training in surgery or medical sub-specialties (such as cardiology) can last as long as 6 to 8 years (compared with 3 for family medicine), the lost earnings from deferring entry into practice for a few years is rapidly recouped. The median compensation of cardiologists, orthopedic surgeons and radiologists in the United States is in excess of $400,000 per year (20% of cardiologists and about 15% or orthopedic surgeons had incomes of more than $600,000 in 2004[10]); gastroenterologists, cancer specialists, eye doctors (opthalmologists) and even dermatologists (the latter are rarely called out of bed in the middle of the night for emergencies) have median incomes of about $320,000; some obviously earn much more depending on the number of procedures they perform.

In addition, many medical students perceive the problem set with which they will deal in PCM as being far more difficult than in the surgical or medical sub-specialties. Consider the following description of a hypothetical medical student observing the practices of a gastroenterologist as compared to a general internist or family practitioner:

> An experienced Gastroenterologist with three assistants guides a colonoscope into a healthy 50-year old man who is comfortably sedated. The physician has performed this procedure thousands of times, and it is routine.
>
> Down the hall, a General Physician, sitting alone in a small exam room, speaks with a frail elderly woman with diabetes, hypertension, atrial fibrillation and asthma, who has recently been hospitalized for gastrointestinal bleeding and now reports extreme fatigue. The physician

must carefully interview the patient to discern what transpired and how she has fared since discharge. Medications to improve her asthma will worsen her diabetes, while drugs that will prevent a stroke caused by the atrial fibrillation could cause the GI bleeding to worsen. A thorough knowledge of the patient's circumstances and conditions is necessary to understand the cause of her symptoms and tailor an effective therapeutic regimen. With only minimal support staff, this physician must gather and integrate a vast amount of information from diverse sources and synthesize the complex medical issues in the personal context of this patient, by weighing anticipated benefits of her 9 prescribed medications against potential adverse effects, considering multiple drug-drug and drug-disease interactions. Then all this must be communicated to the patient in a fashion that a lay person can understand to participate in decision making. . . . In addition to these demanding encounters, the physician devotes several hours each day to data entry, creating detailed documentation, returning phone calls, and completing paperwork for nursing homes, durable medical equipment, disabled parking, and family medical leave.

From the perspective of a trainee, the first physician appears relaxed, content, well supported and amply rewarded. The second is beleaguered, working in isolation poorly supported, and undervalued. It is hardly surprising that the proceduralist is readily perceived as having the more attractive career.[11]

It is little wonder that medical students—despite recruiting efforts specifically designed to augment the number of PCM practitioners—are voting with their feet and entering medical specialties. While few people who make less than a PCM doctor would shed a tear over their income (even taking into account 60 to 70 hour work weeks and very difficult medical problems), the reality is that fewer and fewer students are electing to become primary care providers. There is a general consensus among health care economists and planners that PCMs tend to lower overall medical costs by serving the important functions of minimizing unneeded referrals while at the same time coordinating care among multiple specialists who may not communicate well with each other and thus initiate conflicting treatments that worsen other problems in the organs outside of their specialty. Further, there is virtually uniform agreement that as the population ages the demand for PCM practitioners will increase. Few experts question the need for encouraging newly minted doctors to become primary care providers; yet, so long as 3 to 5 fold disparities in income are in existence, it is difficult to see how recruitment goals for PCM can be achieved.

The disparity in income among medical specialties has been recognized for a long time, and almost two decades ago, an attempt was made to narrow the gap in income. The sad result was that despite efforts to reward physicians based on level of effort and complexity of problems with which they dealt, the income gap hasn't narrowed. It's gotten even wider in the past 15 years. The reasons are predictable (and will probably be no surprise given the information variability of well-reimbursed procedures given earlier in this book): more and more procedures are being done as technology advances, and those procedures are exclusively within the realm of specialists and not primary care providers.

Also reimbursements paid by Medicare and private insurance providers for *procedures* as opposed to *management and evaluation of diseases* (particularly chronic diseases) are much higher on a per hour basis.[12] Since overall cost of any services is a simple product of volume and unit price (in other words, the price per single episode of service), it's no surprise that overall health care costs have grown so quickly and why the lion's share of resources goes to procedurally-oriented specialist physicians who focus their care on something less than the whole patient.

In our view, in private practice specialists are terribly overpaid even when their work hours and deferred compensation from increased training years are taken into account, while primary care physicians are underpaid (but we note that at the VA and in the military, income disparities between specialists and primary care physicians are much smaller and often zero). This view is shared by many if not most health care economists. And while it needn't be this way—specialists in the United Kingdom and other European countries are paid no more than primary care physicians—it seems unlikely that after many years of trying to reverse the trend that there will be a sufficient number of

PCM practitioners. We believe that the solution to the problem is in increasing the number of physician assistants and nurse practitioners in primary care roles.

Increasing the Use of Non-Physician Providers

In 1965, based on his observations of fast-track training of surgical assistants and medics during the Vietnam war, Dr. Eugene Stead of Duke University Medical school introduced the notion of the "physician extender" or "mid-level" health care provider who would work in close concert with physicians to provide much of routine care—both acute and chronic medical management—leaving the physician to deal with more complex cases or unusual diagnostic dilemmas. Dr. Stead's vision was slow to catch on, but after some forty years since the flagship physician-assistant (PA) training program was started at Duke, there are now some 73,000 PAs in the United States. Most have completed an undergraduate college degree and then go on to complete a highly focused two year curriculum in clinical medicine: anatomy, physiology, biochemistry and a full year of working in clinic settings in multiple medical specialties, but largely in primary care.

In similar fashion, the nurse educators realized that many of their students could take courses in addition to the basic nursing curriculum that could qualify them for providing much of routine primary care. There are now in excess of 350,000 nurses with "advanced nursing practice" degrees in the U.S., many working in primary health care services. Unlike PAs who *must* by law be supervised by a physician, in most states nurse practitioners (NPs) can practice independently—literally hanging up their own shingle if they wish—though most elect to work in close collaboration with a physician.

While it is beyond the scope of this book to weigh in on which model provides the best training, there is little doubt that both of these groups of non-physician health care providers (NPHPs) have achieved a high level of acceptance among patients and can do much of primary care.[13] It is no longer unusual for an NPHP to be the first white-coated professional that patients see in clinics, private offices, emergency rooms and urgent care centers, and the decisions they make and services they provide are indistinguishable from those of physicians, at least for the population of patients they serve (who may be, on average, somewhat less complex than patients seen by internists or some family practitioners). While they are well-paid by most people's standards—the median salary of a PA was about $85,000 in 2006—they work hard (average work week of 44 hours), take night call and can, if properly used, dramatically increase the efficiency and economic viability of a primary care office or urgent care center.

And therein lies the rub. Most medical students and residents have worked with NPHPs—they are often on the same hospital rounds or colleagues in ambulatory care environments—but few medical students receive any formal training in how to supervise and /or collaborate with these key health care providers once they start their own practices. We believe that if health care delivery is to be more cost-effective and affordable (no matter how the payment system evolves over time) in the United States, medical resident training, especially in primary care specialties such as general internal medicine and family practice, should include practical instruction on the capabilities of NPHPs and their integration into a collaborative practice in the non-academic setting.

Currently, most primary care physicians do not utilize NPHPs in their practices. But since the overwhelming portion of the health care budget is consumed by management of chronic diseases such as diabetes, coronary artery disease, hypertension, obesity and a few cancer types (any of which could involve specialists at well-chosen times when acute crises supervene) and much of the rest is preventive, episodic or "acute" care for minor illnesses, all of which is within the purview of well-supervised NPHPs, it appears clear that a stronger teaming of physicians with NPHPs is in order. In many individual clinical settings around the country (again the Veterans Administration is the leading example, but federal and state-sponsored Community Health Clinics also apply here), one physician works with between 3 to 5 NPHPs on a regular basis. The NPHPs see more than 80% of the patients—from the very young to the very old—and consult as needed with the physician while the doctor typically sees patients with multiple, interacting medical problems and makes decisions on referrals to specialists, and also receives and analyzes the reports from those specialists.

The evidence supporting the cost-effectiveness of this collaborative practice model—essentially one of a limited number of primary care physicians augmented by a much larger number of NPHPs—is growing rapidly. For example, as just about any doctor will tell you, the management of diabetes in adults is a time-consuming effort and despite the efforts of harried primary care doctors, complication rates of renal failure and coronary artery disease are high. Yet, it is now well known that the frustratingly high rates of complications in this difficult-to-manage patient population is reduced in community health centers.[14] In the challenging context of delivering medical care to the poorest among us who often get treated only when chronic disease has boiled over into a crisis such as a cardiac arrest or heart attack, the same approach is demonstrably successful.[15] The lessons from the collaborative practice model in the Veterans Administration and Community Health Centers should apply well to private-practice and HMO settings. We believe it is well past time to implement them via a carefully structured system of payment incentive and quality review.[16] We outline such a system next.

BRINGING IT ALL TOGETHER: A COMPREHENSIVE UNIFIED SYSTEM OF PAYMENT ("CUSP")

There is no kind way to say it: money drives just about all of healthcare, though there are certainly many health care providers who provide free or minimally reimbursed services in their communities or who volunteer in out-of-the-way, underserved places around the country (and indeed, around the world). However, as we believe the forgoing chapters of this book have made clear, where funding is channeled, so do physicians follow, beginning with the choice of their residency specialty choices when they complete medical school to the practice environments they work in, to the intensity of service that they provide, some of it clearly excessive especially in the procedural oriented specialties.

Thus, if the desirable, long-standing goal of near-universal, affordable health care coverage that is truly responsive to patient needs in the U.S. is to be achieved, a systematic revamping of payment and incentives will be required. Because the best practices in medicine are constantly changing as a result of new technologies and treatments and also constantly updating research findings (often showing that new technologies and treatments aren't nearly as useful as initially though), any rational health care system will have to be dynamic and flexible, that is, changing about as quickly as needs vary and science-based evidence becomes available. We believe that a Comprehensive Uniform System of Payment—CUSP—for the new century must include the following components:

- Rewarding health care providers for preventive care services, including screening for common diseases, vaccination, and counseling for diseases related to life-style choices such as smoking and physical inactivity. Though perhaps mundane on the surface, these interventions are the most cost-effective in all of medical practice.

- Narrowing the income gap among medical specialists. There is no economic justification for cardiologists and radiologists to earn 3 to 5 times as much as a hard working general internist or family practitioner, nor should any physician be earning 15 times the national household income.

- Reducing the wide variation in the use of expensive invasive procedures where the indications or efficacy of those procedures is unclear or unproven. This can be done via payment incentives (or disincentives) and also by rewarding physicians and other health care providers for eliciting patient preferences when choices depend on the patient's tolerance of uncertainty or acceptance of side effects. Contrary to popular belief among physicians, most (though certainly not all) patients can understand the risks and benefits of treatment options and when given the choice, often opt for the least invasive therapies for a variety of common diseases even when those diseases may be life-threatening, such as the most prevalent cancers. And, with non–life threatening conditions that may be painful or debilitating—e.g., degenerative arthritis in the neck or back—most patients are able to weigh the proven benefits of conservative treatments (such as physical therapy) against newer, potentially more beneficial yet riskier treatments (such as surgical fusions). What is clear is that physician preference should never outweigh patient preference.

- Restoring public health as part of medical practice and, at the same time, making medical practice data available to public health officials. Should a serious infectious disease, either naturally-occurring or intentionally introduced via an act of terrorism, break out, with a robust reporting infrastructure to detect the earliest cases, there is good reason to believe that catastrophic consequences can be contained and/or prevented. Yet, for all intents and purposes, the entire country lacks the ability to identify infectious disease outbreaks in their earliest stages. Currently, compliance among physicians for reporting even those diseases they are legally mandated to report is less than 10%. Healthcare providers should be rewarded, again through payment incentives, for participating in reporting of suspected serious infectious disease

- Rewarding physicians for eliciting patient preferences when treatment decisions are ambiguous or of uncertain value.

- Rewarding health care practice—offices, clinics, and hospitals—for doing research based on their own electronic data. Publishing such information is not only desperately needed, it must take place out of the context of the influence of pharmaceutical sponsorship and other biases that skew results (see the example regarding the treatment of insomnia, a very common problem among American adults, below). Publishing results via respected, online "open" journals is now a reality, and while every (or even most) physicians will never take advantage of it, a substantial portion of the practicing health care providers can, bringing the natural experiments—that is, slightly different approaches to treating common medical problems from both the perspective of efficient delivery and effective outcomes—to a huge audience.[17]

- Training more NPHPs (and perhaps producing fewer primary care physicians). NPHPs who have a collaborative relationship with physicians can deliver the bulk of non-surgical and non-procedural health care at a lower cost than physicians alone. We require health manpower studies to determine the most efficient division of labor within the health care system, and then develop long-term incentives to effect a more rational distribution of educational resources.

- Rewarding medical schools for teaching biostatistics and its practical applications in clinical practice—the core of evidence based medicine. No physician should complete their pre-practice training without the ability to read a medical article and interpret the information in light of their own patient population.

- Reduction in overhead costs inherent in the hundreds of insurance companies that collect premiums and distribute them to health care providers. In addition, insurance carriers should be rewarded for sharing information regarding practice patterns of the primary care and subspecialty physicians, physician-assistants, nurse practitioners in order to extract new knowledge for delivering health care efficiently and enhancing ongoing medical education in both disease *and* practice management.

- And finally, rewarding all health care providers and/or the larger systems in which they work for adopting electronic medical records so that compliance with preventive services, best-practice recommendations for the management of chronic disease and medical education can be verified and further enhanced.

CUSP is a form of a "single-payer" health care system. There is a tendency for many medical practitioners and no small number of politicians and editorialists to regard such an approach as "socialized medicine"—where government not only pays for health care but also owns the means for delivering it. But CUSP is, instead, rather akin to a nationwide clearing house of both money *and* information. To be sure, some single-payer systems are indeed government owned and operated medical care—what one finds for the most part, in the United Kingdom and Canada (except of course for rich people who opt out of it altogether, sometimes traveling to other countries to get their health care). But, in other places like Taiwan, a "single payer" system means the government allocates the funds but a myriad of private or semi-private health care delivery systems provide the health care and get paid from one source. In Taiwan, the single-payer system is implemented via a single "smart card" that individuals carry, and much as outlined above, in addition to the easy retrieval of medical records anywhere in the country, exchange of anonymous medical information for research and for internet-based medical education has already been realized.[18]

And, it is not necessary to look to Taiwan or other faraway places for evidence of the efficacy of single-payer strategies that improve access, decrease costs and, amazingly enough, result in better outcomes. For all of the one-off headlines of Canadians who tire of waiting for a procedure or radiologic test (often unnecessary in our view) and come to the U.S. or go elsewhere for care, recent comprehensive reviews give persuasive evidence that for just about any common disease one can name, Canadian patients do better than Americans and at substantially less cost: about half as much per capita as the U.S.,[19] even for difficult problems such as renal failure from diabetes.

There have been and will always be objections to any single-payer system (SPS). Putting aside the faux complaint of looming "socialized medicine," there are understandable grievances about SPSs. As health care economist and Princeton professor Uwe Reinhardt put it in a recent issue of the British Medical Journal[20]:

> Firstly, single-payer systems allocate disproportionate market power to the buy side of health care, which allows government to keep prices at the minimum necessary to keep providers in the system. Providers under-

standably may question the fairness of so asymmetric a distribution of market power in a health system.

To be sure, the low prices it forces on the system allow society to provide more real health care for a given budget than could be delivered in a more expensive pluralistic system and it also makes universal health insurance coverage more affordable. On the other hand, the extremely low profit margins it yields the provider of health care makes single-payer systems less hospitable to innovation in health care products and services and in the organization of health care delivery, areas in which the U.S. excels, sometimes to excess.

Secondly, in single-payer systems spending on health care is pitted against other government priorities and easily falls victim to the politician's perennial desire to campaign on tax cuts. . . . Canada is in the midst of a debate on this issue.

To be "on-the-CUSP" would mean that physicians, the pharmaceutical industry, medication buyers, the research community and, most important, patients themselves would derive the greatest benefit from the ever more seamless flow of information on the best available clinical practices, resulting from "studies" that can be done on data comprising a huge percentage of the population already recorded in charts (electronically, of course). There are a myriad of examples we could add to those already outlined earlier, but we note one more: studies comparing older, generic medications to new medications will never be done simply because the purveyors of the latest medications don't want them to be done and because the manufacturers of generic medications can't afford to fund the study.

Let's take a common problem in adults: insomnia. The vast majority of American adults who complain of inadequate or "non-restorative" sleep don't have conditions like "sleep apnea" (which is all that one ever hears sleep specialists talk about because they can do expensive tests for it in sleep centers) but rather unexplained insomnia. Most end up taking some medication chronically: an anti-depressant perhaps (as many of the members of this class of medication are, in fact, sedating); derivatives of Valium (some long acting, some short acting), or one of the new medications that readers will certainly have seen advertised on television such as Lunestra or Remeron.

The older medications are cheap—literally pennies a night; the newer ones are more than $100 per month. Manufacturers of expensive drugs (who stand to make a lot of money because insomnia rarely goes away, so the drugs are taken chronically) will claim that valium derivatives, while useful initially for the treatment of insomnia, are habit-forming and the patient inevitably requires more and more of the drug to fall asleep. They will also claim that compared to older drugs, their new drugs are both (a) more effective and (b) safer in the long run.

But a comparative study to definitively support or refute those claims has never been done, nor will it ever be. Why? Because the manufacturer of Lunestra doesn't want to take the chance that such a study would show that clonazepam (a long-achieving derivative of valium that costs less than 5 cents per pill) may be neither habit-forming nor require more and more dosage to achieve the same effect or otherwise have any long term side effects as compared to Lunestra. Since there is no requirement from the FDA for a manufacturer to compare a new medication to all existing choices for treating a particular condition, the question is never put to the test.

However, it is highly likely that there are tens of thousand of people taking clonazepam—some for years or decades—who have had no side effects or accelerating dosage requirements. That critical information is buried in their charts, and when statistically compared to patients who are similar in terms of age, sex, and concurrent medical conditions who also have insomnia but are taking the much more expensive Lunestra, one may find that there is no difference in outcome whatsoever (or maybe the patients on clonazepam report even better sleep patterns than the patients taking Lunestra).

One additional clear benefit of any SPS, CUSP included, should be reduction in overhead costs for practitioners and also for payers. There are hundreds of independent hospital and clinic systems and many dozens of large insurance companies across the country. A given physician, physician-assistant or nurse-practitioner may be a member of one health care system—for example, an employee of Kaiser-Permanente in California or Colorado or the Mayo Clinic in Rochester, Minnesota—where he or she practices exclusively, or may contract services to a number of health care systems—for example to several "health maintenance organizations" in a given city or region of a state. Finally, a physician may not be a member or participant in any HMO but instead takes on patients who have "private" insurance such as Blue Cross, "public" insurance such as Medicare or Medicaid or some combination thereof.

Most physicians are not employees of one system (although there is clearly a trend for that happening more and more). Thus, most physicians still have to bill and receive payment from a large number of payers, each with their own forms, electronic reporting requirements, and rules and regulations about what can and can not be done, including, for example, which medication can be prescribed for common conditions like hypertension, heart failure and diabetes. It is a frustrating wilderness of payment plans that confront most doctors and, of course, many patients.

Each of the payers has its own bureaucracy, that is, the staff, building, and consequent overhead in administering its approval and payment processes. There is a cost associated with these individual fiefdoms; most estimates put it at at least 10% of all health care dollars, hardly a small sum when one considers the nation's overall health care bill of around $2.5 trillion dollars (by comparison, Medicare's overhead costs are estimated to be at most 5% of total expenditures, something less than half of what is seen in private practice systems).

But there is an additional "hidden" cost springing from the myriad of payment routes that deserves re-emphasis: each HMO, payer, or unified HMO-payer system shares little, if any of its patient outcome data with anyone else. They are not required to do so. Indeed, only the VA and Medicare regularly report on outcomes, and Medicare is required by law to do so in quite a bit of detail—hence the reason that the Dartmouth study group with whose astounding findings we began this book chose Medicare patients as their "dataset" for identifying the variation in practice patterns and the adverse outcomes associated with that variance across the country. It is difficult for most consumers to understand what value they are receiving for the administrative overhead generated by insurance carriers. While this segment of the health care industry isn't the only one giving questionable return on investment, if the information content gleaned from Medicare by the Dartmouth group or by Veterans Administration directors from their patient data is any guide, insurance companies could easily be part of mitigating rather than further increasing health care costs.

It remains to be seen if the CUSP approach—combining sharing of medical records information among health care providers, medical and public health research, and evaluating physician performance—will be politically acceptable. As a step toward answering this question, we advocate a regional approach in the United States. Large states or groupings of smaller states could set up their own CUSPs with varying implementations of the research, education, and payment functions of the CUSP though with a uniform structure for electronic medical records. In this manner, a few variations-on-the-theme can be tested and either proven or rejected. We believe that given the successes of the single-payer methods in other countries that it is unlikely that a style suitable to the overwhelming majority of Americans can be found, while at the same time increasing the satisfaction of primary care physicians and their NPHP colleagues.

In short, CUSP offers an exchange to the many players and payers in the health care system: rapid, reliable, payment for services with minimal bureaucratic overhead and wasted time in exchange for real-world practice information that will further reduce costs allowing more people without insurance to receive it. And with this information will come new guidelines for common conditions—and the all-too-common complications when several common conditions obtain in the same patient. We believe that it is even likely that burdensome lawsuits from doing either "too little" or "too much" can be minimized as health care providers learn about their own practice habits and how they comport with best practice recommendations and evidence-based medicine that is at their fingertips.

A single payer system like CUSP, which combines the functions of reimbursing health care providers with continuous monitoring of disease patterns and practice variations and the provision feedback to physicians and NPHPs to reinforce high quality shared decision-making with patients is achievable and is, in our view, the best possible opportunity to slow or even reverse health care cost inflation in the

U.S., making near universal coverage affordable, practical, and truly beneficial to just about everyone. In the U.S. polity, no one can be forced to practice under such a system nor can every patient be compelled to receive their health care from it; there will always be a few people who can afford to purchase as much health care as they want (even if the evidence continues to show that such choices do more harm than good) and there will always be physicians willing to provide it. But the opportunities for cost reduction under a CUSP may be so large as to all but marginalize the latter.

Some risks are worth taking.

NOTES

1. For a more detailed discussion on why the current worry about avian influenza in humans is probably overblown, see: Zelicoff, A. P. "Avian Influenza," February 2007, available on-line at: http://www.zelicoff.com/InfluenzaWhitePaperv2a.pdf.
2. K. Eban, "Biosense or biononsense?" *Scientist*, April 2007; vol 21 (4), pp. 32–38.
3. http://www.medschool.pitt.edu/PDFs/06–07%20Fact%20Book-published%20version.pdf.
4. C.P. West and R.D Ficolora, "Clinician Attitudes Toward Biostatistics," Mayo Clinic Proceedings, 82(8): 939–43, 2007.
5. http://services.aamc.org/currdir/start.cfm.
6. http://services.aamc.org/currdir/section2/04_05hottopics.pdf.
7. D.M. Windish, S.J. Huot, and M.L. Green, "Medicine Residents' Understanding of the Biostatistics and Results in the Medical Literature," *Journal of the American Medical Association* (2007) vol. 298(9), pp. 1010–1023.
8. The Clinical Guideline to Preventive Services, Recommendations of the U.S. Preventive Services Task Forces (USPSTF) and the Agency for Healthcare Research and Quality(AHRQ) 2006, http://www.ahrq.gov/clinic/prevenix.htm (free pocketguide available); U.S. Preventive Services Task Force (USPSTF) *Guide to Clinical Preventive Services*, 2nd ed., Williams and Wilkins 1996.
9. T. Bodenheimer, R.A. Berenson, and P. Rudolf, "The Primary Care-Specialty Income Gap: Why it Matters," *Annals of Internal Medicine*, 2007 l 146: pp. 301–306.
10. R. Lowes, "The earnings freeze. Now it's everybody's problem." *Med Econ.*, 2005;82:58–62, 64, 66–8.
11. Blue Ribbon Panel of the Society of General Internal Medicine. Redesigning the Practice Model for General Internal Medicine. A Proposal for Coordinated Care. A Policy Monograph of the Society of General Internal Medicine. Journal of General Internal Medicine, vol. 22(3), 2007, pp. 400–409.
12. G.F. Anderson, U.E. Reinhardt, and V. Petrosyan, "It's the Prices, Stupid: Why the United States Is So Different from Other Countries," *Health Affairs*, vol. 22(3) 2003, pp.. 89–105.
13. D.W. Roblin, E.R. Becker, E.K. Adams, D.H. Howard, and M.H. Roberts, "Patient

satisfaction with primary care: does type of practitioner matter?" *Med Care*, June 2004, 42(6):579–90.

14. E.S. Huang, Q. Zhang, S.E. Brown, M.L. Drum, D.O. Meltzer, and M.H. Chin, D.O., Chin, "The cost-effectiveness of improving diabetes care in U.S. Federally qualified community health centers," *Health Serv. Res.* December 2007, 42(6 Pt 1):2174–93.

15. M. Proser, "Deserving the spotlight: health centers provide high-quality and cost-effective care," *J Ambul Care Manage*, October–December 2005, 28(4):321–30.

16. D. Hawkins and S. Rosenbaum, "Health centers at 40: implications for future public policy," *J Ambul Care Manage*, October–December 2005, 28(4):357–65.

17. J. Willinsky, S. Murray, C. Kendall, and A. Palepu, "Doing medical journals differently: open medicine, open access and academic freedom," *Can J Commun*, 2007, http://pkp.sfu.ca/node/776. (last accessed Jan 2, 2008); see also: Dean Giustini, "Web 3.0 and medicine," *British Medical Journal*, vol. 335, 2007, pp. 1273–4.

18. W.H. Tsai and K.C. Kuo, *International Journal of Electronic Healthcare*, 2007;3(4):417–32. The internet and health care in Taiwan: value-added applications on the medical network in the National Health Insurance smart card system.

19. Gordon H. Guyatt, P.J. Devereaux, Joel Lexchin, et al. "A systematic review of studies comparing health outcomes in Canada and the United States," *Open Medicine*, 2007;1(1):e27–36.

20. U.E. Reinhardt, "Single-payer systems spark endless debate—Are they a panacea or a form of 'socialised medicine'? Americans just cannot agree," *British Medical Journal*, April 28, 2007; v.334, no.7599, p.881.

INDEX